Immigrant Women and Their Health:

an olive paper

D1522623

Afaf Ibrahim Meleis
Juliene G. Lipson
Marjorie Muecke
Gloria Smith

Sigma Theta Tau International
Center Nursing Press
550 West North Street
Indianapolis, Indiana 46202

Sigma Theta Tau International
Center Nursing Press
Peer-reviewed Publications

Date	Title
1992	Leonard Felix Fuld, 19th Century Reformer in a 20th Century World
1997	The Image Editors: Mind, Spirit, and Voice
1997	The Language of Nursing Theory and Metatheory
1997	The Adventurous Years: Leaders in Action, 1973-1993, a Nell Watts memoir
1997	Virginia Avenel Henderson: Signature for Nursing
1998	The Neuman Systems Model and Nursing Education: Teaching Strategies and Outcomes

For other Center Nursing Press publications and videos, contact:
Sigma Theta Tau International
550 West North Street
Indianapolis, IN 46202
1.888.634.7575
FAX: 317.634.8188
www.stti.iupui.edu

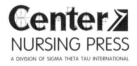

Center
NURSING PRESS
A DIVISION OF SIGMA THETA TAU INTERNATIONAL

ISBN: 0-9656391-6-9

Printed in the United States of America

Views expressed herein are not necessarily
those of Sigma Theta Tau International.

Table of Contents

Appendix A:
Culturally Appropriate Programs for Immigrant Women: Exemplars .. 44

Appendix B:

Authors

Afaf Ibrahim Meleis, RN, PhD, FAAN
Professor
University of California
San Francisco

Juliene G. Lipson, RN, PhD, FAAN
Professor
University of California
San Francisco

Marjorie Muecke, RN, PhD, FAAN
Program Officer
The Ford Foundation
and Professor
University of Washington

Gloria Smith, RN, PhD, FAAN
Vice-President
W.K. Kellogg Foundation

Originally prepared for "Health Care in Time of Global Transition," an Annual Meeting of The American Academy of Nursing, November 9-12, 1995, Washington, DC.

FOREWORD

Immigrant Women and Their Health: An Olive Paper

Migration and population relocation are part of human history. However, recent national and international issues create a need to pay more attention to immigration and its effects on immigrants and the societies in which immigrants resettle. Women constitute about 80% of the world's total of immigrants and refugees. Women immigrants are less visible than are men immigrants. They often receive less health care and care of inferior quality; and they have received less scholarly attention. As a result their health may be compromised.

The overall goal of this paper, which we are calling an olive paper,[1] is to raise nurses' consciousness about the urgent need to address health care issues of immigrants in general and immigrant women in particular.[2] We hope that leaders in nursing practice, education, research, and administration will review this document. We also believe that it will be of interdisciplinary interest. Those providing health care to minority, marginalized, and diverse populations, as well as those with interest in culture and health, may find this monograph helpful. It is also intended for policy makers and for state and national legislators. Therefore, the authors' overall goal is to stimulate interest in dialogue about these issues and, in turn, to prepare readers to influence policy makers to improve health care for immigrant women.

---

[1]The authors of this olive paper question the assumption that important policy papers should be "white," especially when many of the women who are the focus of this paper have olive-colored skin.

[2]We use the word immigrant to encompass such categories as voluntary immigrant, forced immigrant, undocumented immigrant, and refugee. While reasons for choosing or being forced to leave one's home country differ, the issues associated with health and with living in a host country are quite similar.

Specifically, the purposes of this monograph are to (a) establish a framework that describes the issues and risks that compromise immigrant women's health and health care, safety, human rights, self-sufficiency, and contributions; (b) identify models of excellence in providing immigrant women with equitable and culturally competent health care; (c) analyze principles that ensure the provision of culturally competent care for immigrant women; and (d) identify recommendations, strategies, and priorities to guide policy dialogues to ensure immigrant women's access to and utilization of high-quality health care to enhance their wellness and safety.

SECTION

I.

Background, Context, and Analytic Framework

The social climate of the United States in the 1990s is confusing for immigrants and presents difficulties concerning health care delivery. At this time, it is particularly important to focus on health needs of first-generation foreign-born people because of widespread xenophobia expressed in the public communications media and political arenas. During times of economic recession and corporate downsizing, conservative ideologies increase in influence—tending to stereotype women and disenfranchise them even more (Faludi, 1991). This social and political environment increases the health risks of women. Immigrant women tend to work in small shops and at jobs that provide limited or no benefits, such as housecleaning and child care (Tienda, Jensen, & Bach, 1984). Their vulnerability is increased by their work conditions and poverty and by society's anti-women, anti-immigrant bias. Some immigrant women's visas are temporary or their status is undocumented, adding another source of vulnerability.

Immigrant and refugee women are similar to other minority women who are vulnerable to ill health and poor-quality lifestyle *because they are women*, because they *have different explanatory frameworks of illness*, because they *are in transition*, and because they *are marginalized* (Meleis, 1995). We organize these concerns using Meleis' framework for analysis of immigrant women's health care in developed countries (Meleis, 1995). The framework has four parts: gender and health, explanatory models of illness, transitions and health, and marginalization.

Gender and Health

Examination of the literature on women's health care reveals common neglected themes that transcend geographic location and immigration status, as well as those specific to cultural and socioeconomic contexts. Women all over the world have been viewed mainly in terms of their reproductive needs and abilities, with scant attention paid to understanding, diagnosing, and preventing health problems related to gender. We have recently recognized, however, that women's health care needs go beyond pregnancy and childbearing. For example, while cardiovascular disease is a leading cause of death for both men and women, decisions related to diagnoses, risk factors, and prevention for women are based on decades of research done on men; women with cardiovascular diseases tend to be ignored, misdiagnosed, or diagnosed late (Rankin, 1989).

Recent research findings on women and heart disease are based on pooling small samples from male-dominated studies; and large-scale prospective studies such as the Women's Health Initiative have just recently begun (Flavell, 1994). An urgent need also exists to understand health risks unique or more prevalent among women, for example, gallstones and urinary incontinence. Breast cancer, osteoporosis, and depression related to menopausal transition are primarily women's conditions; girls and women comprise most of the victims of rape, sexual abuse, and domestic violence (Heiss, Patting, & Germaine, 1994). Furthermore, issues related to women's aging, coping with second careers, and self-care activities have either been ignored or received minimal attention.

Research with immigrant and refugee women reflects the same imbalance, particularly the focus on women as reproductive rather than productive beings. Kulig's (1990) review of research on Southeast Asian refugee women revealed that the majority of studies focused on women's childbearing role, emphasizing their related cultural beliefs and implications for the health care delivery system. As a result, knowledge about health and health needs as perceived by these women is still very limited. While cardiovascular disease is the largest killer of Latina women in the United States, almost no studies of women's risk factors have been published (Juarbe, 1996).

Women in general are disadvantaged in the job market; the relationship between their economic well being and overall health needs has been inadequately considered (Stier, 1991). Women are also the main caregivers in families and communities, and although they typically have multiple roles simultaneously, their health needs related to these roles have not been fully examined (Meleis, Norbeck, Laffrey, Solomon, & Miller, 1989).

Women are also vulnerable to violence because they are women. Gender-based violence against women including rape, domestic violence, mutilation, sexual abuse, and murder is a major health problem for women worldwide (Heiss, Patting, & Germaine, 1994). Immigrant or "translocated" women are even more vulnerable in this regard (Ogur, 1990). Many immigrant women have survived politically motivated violence or sexual aggression in their home country (Amnesty International, 1995) or during their immigration journey. They are reluctant to speak up about violent acts for the same reasons that native-born women are reluctant to disclose rape, sexual abuse, and sexual harassment. In addition, immigrant women may be more reluctant to report such incidents for fear of being deported, stereotyped, and even more isolated.

Work roles raise health-related issues for immigrant women. In most cases, work outside the home increases their power base within their families and communities and improves their domestic social relations. However, such work sometimes creates marital disharmony, particularly in couples from patrilineally organized societies, because outside employment increases women's social and economic freedom and independence (Lipson & Miller, 1994). However, often this new autonomy seems not to raise their consciousness or willingness to initiate changes in their work situations. Pessar (1984) concludes that family value systems, beliefs about the goals of immigration, and daily stressors associated with function in a new country tend to reduce immigrants' identification with other workers and to decrease their willingness to organize to institute changes. Because most are working very hard in a new environment, they are simply too drained of physical and emotional resources to participate in collective activities.

Explanatory Models of Illness

Indications are strong that women's cognitive styles differ from men's (Gilligan, 1982). Immigrant women in particular also tend to have explanatory models of illness, disease, and health that are different from those of the dominant European-American society and from the biomedical system (Kleinman, 1980). Without knowledge about these perspectives, health care professionals cannot understand the experiences and meanings for individuals and may make inappropriate clinical judgments. For example, immigrant Chinese women were shown vignettes depicting depression and asked to conceptualize the problem and to state causes, potential effects on individuals, and potential sources of help (Ying, 1990). Those who conceptualized depression as physical tended to suggest that the person should seek medical services. However, those who conceptualized depression as a psychological condition tended to suggest that the depressed individual should seek help from family and friends rather than professionals. Yet, because families are not always the best resources for meeting women's mental health needs and may even blame them for their depression, these women often do not get the help they need.

Cultural heritage, norms, and values provide people with explanatory frameworks and guide them in choosing one model of treatment over another. Immigrant women tend to use culturally-based health care sources and often wait to seek help from biomedical professionals until all their customary practices in taking care of themselves are exhausted. Acculturation levels do not consistently predict when, how, or from whom they seek health care (Van der Stuyft, De Muynck, Schillemans, & Timmerman, 1989). The variety of patterns of health care utilization are not well documented in the literature. As our goal is to support these patterns or enhance them, health promotion and utilization practices must be carefully examined and described (Sanders-Phillips, 1994).

Transitions and Health

Times of transition are periods during which people perceive change to be occurring in a person or the environment in which the person functions (Chick & Meleis, 1986). Transitions of immigration resettlement are prime examples of significant changes in both people and environment. During transitions, immigrant women have numerous roles, such as maintaining ethnic continuity. They are the culture brokers and family mediators. Their immediate and extended families typically expect them to maintain their culture of origin, help family members maintain it, and, at the same time, help family members integrate into the educational and social systems of society (Hattar-Pollara & Meleis, 1995a; Hattar-Pollara & Meleis, 1995b). This double burden is added to their role overload of other responsibilities that include taking care of extended family locally and abroad (Meleis, 1991).

The immigrants' transition imposes other burdens. Aroian's (1990) study of Polish immigrants in the United States identified such immigration-based stressors as the novelty of the new environment, occupation, and language; not "feeling at home"; and the feeling of being subordinate in the host society. Stressors experienced by Iranian women immigrants include occupational and financial difficulties, loss of status, reduced social support, ethnic bias, and differences in values and child rearing styles (Lipson, 1992). A major stressor experienced by a Lao community in Seattle was the threat of persecution by an evil spirit from the home country for having fled home, kind, and country (Muecke, 1987).

During transition periods there is often loss of support until new support systems are established; since social support is one of the major variables linked to physical and mental health, health may be compromised. In the immigrant transition, immigrants' friends and support system are frequently their relatives; if the relatives live in another city or country, immigrant women suffer because support is limited. While women in many countries consider their adult children a source of support (see, for example, Meleis & Bernal, 1996; Meleis, Douglas, Eribes, Shih, & Messias, 1996), it is interesting that in one study, Mexican immigrant women did not (Vega, Kolody, Valle, & Weir, 1991). Thus, the nature of family support should receive more scholarly attention. Having a social network does not always provide support for immigrant women; it is important for health that the network provide emotional support (Vega, Kolody, Valle, & Hough, 1986).

Immigrant women are also faced with a new society, new values, new norms, and new sets of expectations. Confrontation by so much that is new tends to create a sense of disequilibrium and uncertainty. Transitions may also evoke fear of identity loss or changes in roles, patterns of behavior, and dynamics of interaction (Schumacher & Meleis, 1994). In one study in which the majority of participants were from minority groups or were immigrants, women's stories demonstrated an increased sense of vulnerability during times of transition. Women described feeling torn away from a familiar and established pattern and put in a setting for which they felt unprepared emotionally and culturally (Stevens, Hall, & Meleis, 1992). These feelings of uprootedness, coupled with the need to function in an unfamiliar environment in which the symbols have to be constantly interpreted, led to these women feeling distress manifested as depression and somatic complaints (Mirdal, 1984). This distress added to their feeling of isolation and the perception that they were not well understood. A theme of persistent grief may influence everything in the life of immigrant women (Anderson, 1991).

Effects of life transitions may be cumulative. If issues related to one transition are not resolved, they may be aggravated when another transition arises. This cumulative effect results in a different meaning and experience for immigrant women from that of nonimmigrant women. The postpartum transition, for example, added to an immigration transition, results in changes in social roles, lifestyle, interaction, and support system. Women going through both transitions simultaneously have distinct issues, for example, a constant appraisal of uncertainties, conflicts between traditional and modern systems of birth, and postpartum strain (El Sayed, 1986).

Transitions also intersect with health status. For immigrant women, problems of living with a chronic illness are compounded by feelings of being "uprooted" (Anderson, 1991). Women migrant farm workers who are constantly relocating are often vulnerable to tuberculosis and urinary tract infections (Bechtel, Shepherd, & Rogers, 1995). There is a strong association between depression and resettlement and between mental illness and the refugee experience, particularly among those who were exposed to persecution and who endured many years of camp life (Franks & Faux, 1990). Therefore, health care for immigrant women must take all their transitions into account as a context for the total assessment of their needs and for developing knowledge on which to base intervention strategies.

Marginalization and Health

Immigrant women share many issues that confront many minority women and women of color in particular. Their accents or appearance often set them apart in the eyes of people of the dominant culture, who may treat them with disrespect, much as minority women are often set apart and treated with low regard or even virulent prejudice (Lalonde, Taylor, & Moghaddam, 1992).

Immigrant women often have to deal with unfriendly neighbors and outright hostility in their immediate communities. Many are frustrated and saddened by constant reminders that they do not belong, which makes their integration into the mainstream even more difficult (Hattar-Pollara & Meleis, 1995a).

Immigrant women are vulnerable when they are marginalized by main-stream society on the basis of perceived differences. Marginalization is defined as being different in the sense of being negatively distinguished from the norm. Margins are defined as "the peripheral, boundary-determining aspects of persons, social networks, communities, and environments" (Hall, Stevens, & Meleis, 1994, pp. 24-25). Marginalized people react and respond to situations in ways mainstream people consider unique or odd. They may be distinguished by their dress, language, religious practices, food preferences, or other characteristics. Marginalization increases as the person or group moves farther away from practices of those at the center. The center is determined by the majority and populated by more powerful mainstream people. Marginalized people are allowed little power, and their strengths tend not to be understood by the majority of people. While the power of people at the periphery is constantly challenged and denied, the power of people at the center is usually uncontested. Under these circumstances, marginalized people learn to be secretive and to guard information that may expose their marginalization or further marginalize them. They learn to disclose personal information only to those with whom they have developed trust and feel safe. Although they tend to be more reflective about their own and others' behavior and often have profound insights, they may appear silent and voiceless. All these characteristics set them apart and thus marginalize them even more.

Women immigrants with low-income, with low-status jobs, or receiving public aid share the problems of marginalization that confront other impoverished women. The largest percentage of women workers occupy lower status jobs, and immigrant women tend to have jobs with low status (Boyd, 1984). In addition to dead-end, low-status, and low-prestige occupations such as domestic work, grocery store attendant, or fast-food clerk, women often work triple shifts in their daily lives (Lipson & Miller, 1994; Nelson, 1995). For economic reasons, many take two jobs and, in addition, are homemakers; many care for other relatives. They are minimally compensated, and in some instances, they have limited control over the money they earn. Because much of their work is informal, it is not reflected in statistics, and the women are considered nonproductive. We suspect that immigrants from European countries have better job opportunities than those from developing countries. There has been minimal examination of workplace conditions in jobs held predominantly by women. For example, immigrants often work in situations that tend to oppress them more, an issue that must be uncovered, examined, and discussed.

Immigrant women are marginalized in health care as well. Even in the Scandinavian countries, considered models of equity and fairness, there are differences in the way natives and foreign-born patients are treated. In a Swedish study, investigators found that, compared with nonimmigrant

Swedes, immigrants tended to use hospital emergency departments more and hospital outpatient departments less often and are less well integrated into mainstream health care (Magnusson & Aurelius, 1980). Immigrants in the United States tend to receive more fragmented care than native-born people, a situation that often leads to more emergency care. In one group of immigrant women, 20% of hospital admissions were due to undiagnosed or poorly defined causes. The authors concluded that there are institutional barriers that make access a problem for immigrants. These barriers tend to further marginalize women and immigrants.

Because of their marginalization, immigrants tend to feel stereotyped, misunderstood, and set apart. Therefore, they tend to work hard at creating a more familiar atmosphere in which they can relate to other people by finding some common ground. Although this takes time and energy, it demonstrates resilience. However, people in host societies are often not sufficiently patient to accommodate the time it takes to find common ground.

Social values that determine who is marginalized influence the philosophy upon which education and health care systems are built. Therefore, it is not enough to make changes in the health care system and to strive to provide structurally competent care. Health care professionals must strive to make some fundamental changes in the dominant ideologies in training institutions and in societies (Anderson, 1987; Jones, 1988).

SECTION

II.

Health Care Issues

The health care issues of immigrant women reflect their social marginalization and their newness to our society. They often present their perceptions of symptoms using frameworks that are not well understood by providers. Many have little or no time for stress-reducing activities or regular exercise. Many adopt readily available, unhealthy diets promoted by the U.S. communications media; they have little access to health education to help them incorporate the healthy aspects of their traditional diets. Their daily worries, such as fear of deportation, which undermine their willingness to report incidents of domestic violence, may compromise their health. Mental health resources are limited and fail to acknowledge their similarities and differences.

We identified four types of health-care issues that have implications for health care policy relevant to immigrant women: poor definition as a population; vulnerability to health risks including mental-health risks; barriers to health care; and under-recognition of resources.

Immigrant Women are not Well Defined as a Population

The diversity of immigrant women may be a deterrent to developing useful research frameworks to guide culturally competent health care. "Immigrant" is a broad category that includes many people with unique needs and diverse health care issues. In the literature, researchers describe several variables that influence the definition of immigrants and refugee women, such as time in the United States, immigrant or refugee status, voluntary or forced immigration, and current political relationships between the home country and the United States. When a woman stops being an "immigrant" is not clear.

Other concerns center on inclusion of women immigrants in clinical studies about providing women's health care. Above, we mentioned the tendency to focus exclusively on women's childbearing function. Unfortunately, women's health has had limited attention from scholars about the broad health care issues encountered by immigrant women.

Immigrant Women are Vulnerable to Health Risks

The increased vulnerability of immigrant women to health risks is related to their gender and the context of their experiences of immigration. For example, immigration itself has been associated with increased morbidity, such as classic studies demonstrating different rates of coronary heart disease and stroke in Japanese men in Japan, Hawaii, and California (Kagan, Harris, Winkelstein, Johnson, & Kato, 1974). "Acculturation" broadly defined, but signifying assimilation into U.S. lifestyle patterns, has been associated frequently with increased morbidity among Hispanics (Castro, Baezconde-Garbanati, & Beltran, 1985). United States-oriented women have been found to have significantly higher risk of delivering low-birth-weight infants than Mexican-oriented women (Scribner & Dwyer, 1989). More recently, emphasis on greater use of English versus Spanish language among Hispanic women has dominated in studies of acculturation effects on low-birth-weight status (Cobas, Balcazar, Benin, Keith, & Chong, 1996).

Some risks might be unrecognized or poorly understood by health care professionals. For example, women from the Middle East with schistosomiasis and women who develop prolapsed uterus who come from societies that encourage large numbers of children may be misdiagnosed, undiscovered, or medically mismanaged. Health risks may be increased for women who have no access to health education in a culturally appropriate format or language. Thus, they may not understand the reasons for preventive health care or such concerns as diet and exercise. For example, Lipson, Hosseini, Kabir, Omidian, and Edmonston (1995) found that Afghan refugee women knew little about their anatomy—for example, what a kidney or bladder is, nor about such physiologic processes as menstruation or menopause. Sex-education classes in Afghanistan and Pakistan were nonexistent because such information was thought to encourage promiscuity; it was also too embarrassing a subject to discuss even with close female family members and friends. In the less socially constrained United States, lack of information puts some young Afghan women at risk for pregnancy and sexually transmitted disease when their parents prohibit taking high school sex-education classes.

Immigrant women are at high risk for domestic violence. They tend to be silent about it because of family values of loyalty or for fear of deportation and further aggression. Researchers in California found that 48% of Latina women reporting violence indicated that such violence had increased in intensity since moving to the United States (National Council for Research on Women, 1995). Women immigrants are also at risk for stress-related physical symptoms and mental health problems because of a combination of such factors as multiple roles and responsibilities, language problems, culture conflict, economic and occupational stressors, negative public attitudes, traumatic experiences in the country of origin, and perceived lack of social support. The best predictors of depression among Mexican immigrant women are lack of family support and low income (Vega, Kolody, & Valle, 1987; Vega et al., 1991).

Barriers to Care

Immigrant women have the same health care access problems as other minority and marginalized women, such as having no health insurance and little money to pay for health care. Further, their health care providers may be unaware of differences in world view or explanatory models of illness or other pertinent realities of these women's everyday lives. Immigrant women may seek care only when very ill because their employers do not provide sick leave, dock their pay, or threaten termination if the worker should seek care during daytime work hours when most clinics are open. Immigrant women also have time limitations because of the nature and extent of their responsibilities, their work, and demands of their extended families.

They face the daunting complexity of learning how to access health care services and dealing with language barriers. Inadequate English interferes with identifying an appropriate source for care, making appointments, describing one's problem, and understanding verbal and written instructions. Simply finding a family or friend with sufficient time and English-speaking ability to accompany and interpret may be daunting enough to discourage care-seeking except for emergencies (Lipson & Omidian, 1997). Communication issues are described further in the section on principles for culturally competent care.

Typically, there are few culturally appropriate care contexts and no or limited outreach and health education programs for immigrant women, except in some areas in which the immigrant population is large (see Appendix A, Programs 2 and 5). All these factors influence and limit women's access to high-quality health care.

Immigrant Women are Unrecognized Resources

The fourth set of issues stems from lack of recognition and understanding of immigrant women's inner resources and power. Service providers regard power from a Western perspective, for example, being vocal, assertive, and other behavior specific to Euro-American culture. However, the power of some immigrant women is derived from their maternal roles, involvement in family business, or support of extended family. Further, the biomedical perspective often guides health researchers and practitioners to focus on pathology rather than on factors facilitating health.

Nevertheless, at least a few studies identify healthy practices among immigrants. For example, a comparative study conducted in Seattle among Hmong and Vietnamese refugees and women born in this country found that not smoking and avoidance of beverage alcohol were protective factors contributing to healthy birth outcomes (Hahn & Muecke, 1987).

Much of the literature on immigration addresses the pathologic influence of migration, paying little attention to those who succeed in relocating (Muecke, 1992). A major question is whether immigrants are inherently hardier than nonimmigrants of the same national and ethnic origin. Aroian (1990) criticizes both the use of static outcome measures of psychological functioning unrelated to the sources of distress and the tendency to view migration only as a risk. Her study of Polish immigrants and Rumbaut's (1985) study of psychological adjustment among Southeast Asian refugees examine both "pathogenesis" and "salutogenesis" (Antonovsky, 1979), the latter signifying use of adaptive resources and successful coping amidst ubiquitous stressors. In other words, it may be the hardiest who choose to immigrate or who survive the conditions that lead to their becoming refugees.

Similarly, there is little research on genetic resources that may buffer immigrant women from illness. There are some indications that foreign-born immigrants tend to do much better on some health indicators than non-foreign-born people. For example, the infants of immigrant Hispanic women are larger and healthier than those of Hispanic women born in the United States (Mendoza, Ventura, Burciaga-Valdez, Castillo, Escoto Saldiva, Baisden, & Martorell, 1991).

Finally, there is a need for more research that incorporates the immigrants' cultural idiom of healthy behaviors and beliefs. For example, Thompson (1991) examined symbolic traditions that Cambodian women brought with them to the United States as a means of reconfirming with them their stories of women's strength and resistance to oppression.

Culturally Appropriate Health Care: Exemplars

We identified 10 exemplary programs that were specifically designed to provide health care for immigrant women and describe them briefly in Appendix A. These programs were developed using a variety of criteria to ensure that they are culturally appropriate. Most relied heavily on immigrant community input and participation to meet needs identified by the community or multi-cultural population. Some of the programs have lasted a long time because of ongoing fundraising efforts of a cadre of dedicated volunteers and strong community support, while others have been discontinued for lack of funding. There is no single source of information about such programs and most of them are not described in the published scholarly literature. From our review of a number of sources and on use of our personal contacts, we selected a convenience sample of exemplar programs. We identified four types of exemplary programs based on who initiated them—service agency, community, individual nurse, or professional nursing association. Some programs fit more than one category. These categories are not intended to be comprehensive or mutually exclusive, nor are exclusions intentional.

Health or Social Service Agency Programs

These programs were developed by mainstream health care or social service agencies and are supported by city, state, or federal funding or by foundation grants. They may have been initiated with a foundation grant and may or may not have received later support from an institution. Staff is often comprised of regular agency personnel and those hired specifically for the project. The group is usually multinational—in many instances multicultural—or has specific cultural training reflecting the cultural and language backgrounds of the populations served.

These programs include those that are provided to a group of women for an identified problem and those that are in partnership with other agencies or community representatives to provide services. Examples are Programs 1, 2, and 3.

Community-Initiated Programs

These programs are initiated by community members and usually remain within community control. Funding may be sought through government agencies, foundations, or private organizations—and the community itself provides volunteers and donations. These programs tend to provide comprehensive services based on the expressed needs of community members and grounded in the culture of the participants. Some programs meet a variety of health needs through their activities, even when they do not specifically focus on health. Program 3 partially exemplifies this category, as do Programs 4, 5, and 6.

Nurse-Initiated Programs

These programs were developed by nurses who identified the health care needs of a particular population in a community and designed special programs to meet these needs. Such programs are funded through many sources including private foundations, government service and research grants, and funds provided by the community. While developed and staffed by nurses, such programs succeed because of community partnership, use of volunteers, and cooperation among all interested groups. Programs rely heavily on the resources already presented in the community. An excellent example is the De Madres A Madres program developed by a community health nurse who established a community partnership to provide social support and information to encourage Hispanic women to begin early prenatal care (Mahon, McFarlane, & Golden, 1991). Programs 6, 7, 8, and 9 are other examples.

Professional Nursing Organizations

Professional nursing organizations have developed culturally competent health programs for specific immigrant community needs, either singly as one organization, as described in Program 10 in Appendix A, or through participating in a coalition of organizations such as the National Coalition of Hispanic Health and Human Service Organizations (COSSMHO) or the National Black Women's Health Project of Washington, DC.

Culturally Competent Health Care Programs for Immigrant Women: Principles

Culturally competent care has been defined as care that is sensitive to issues related to culture, race, gender, sexual orientation, explanatory frameworks, transitions, marginalization, and financial situation (Meleis, Isenberg, Koerner, & Stern, 1995). To provide culturally competent care to immigrant women, their presence, their experiences, and their worldview should be acknowledged both by society and health care providers.

Immigrant women share inequalities experienced by all women—inequalities in education, work, and health care. They also share problems associated with limited scholarly attention being paid to their unique health problems, with access to care, exposure to and ill effects of violence, and health problems of old age, such as osteoporosis and cardiovascular disease. However, immigrant women are distinctive in their perspective, their explanatory frameworks of health and illness, their transition experiences, and their marginalization. Because they are often overworked and often focus mainly on resettlement and economic survival, they tend to be isolated from the host community. They may also be isolated by gender inequities and by the dominance of men in their lives. Isolation itself can disempower. People in the dominant society usually tend to make immigrant women voiceless, keep them at arm's length, stereotype them, and distinguish them by their differences. Emphasis on language barriers, accents, clothing, and color of skin marginalizes them even more.

Many immigrant women have, however, become more resilient through having faced and adapted to many challenges and by becoming bicultural. While transition experiences are painful, they also stimulate growth and transformation. These experiences should be described and addressed. Issues related to gender, explanatory frameworks, transitions, and marginalization act as barriers to access to health care, to protective health behaviors, and to the experience of better health. As health care professionals, we have knowledge in these areas useful in providing good health care for women immigrants.

We suggest the following conditions for providing immigrant women with culturally competent care[3]. First, their health should be considered within the context of their diversity. Second, a gender-based perspective should be used as a framework for understanding women's situations and particularly for focusing on women's multiple roles. Third, transition is an important framework for considering immigrant women's experiences. Fourth, we must critically consider how the current dominant society's ideology, climate, and prevailing value systems frame education and health care services. We must consider whether these factors marginalize women and how such marginalization could in turn influence their daily lives. However, these suggestions will be ineffective unless we confront our own biases. Therefore, fifth, we must begin by being in touch with our own values, ideologies, and stereotyping behaviors.

While several strategies have been used to promote culturally competent care, we need to develop and test many more (Meleis, Isenberg, Koerner, & Stern, 1995). Two examples of strategies are cultural brokerage that interprets language and culture (Barbee, 1987; Budman, Lipson, & Meleis, 1992; Jezewski, 1990; Tripp-Reimer & Brink, 1984) and provision of somatic care even when mental health care is required (Flaskerud, 1987).

The exemplars mentioned in this monograph and summarized in Appendix A have a number of characteristics in common. All the programs focus on women and their situations. They are designed with consideration for women's perspectives, subjective experiences, cultural heritage, and transitions experiences. Principles that should underlie the design and development of culturally competent programs for immigrant women are uniqueness, flexible use of time, provision of comprehensive personal services, and empowerment.

Uniqueness

A culturally competent program should be built on the unique needs, resources, and practices of the population for which it is developed. For example, knowing that survivors of the Khmer Rouge regime may not be able to verbalize their trauma and recognizing the significance of these experiences in the lives of those who endured them, three innovative programs (see Programs 1, 3, and 4) were developed to help the women deal with their post-traumatic stress disorder. An experienced Cambodian community-clinic interpreter developed a group in which women could come together to sew quilts. The women worked silently at first but gradually made informal comments that developed into conversations. Conversations progressed to sharing of experiences and finally enough trust was developed to permit relationships with the clinic staff. A nurse-researcher devel-

---

[3]We recognize that the concept, culturally competent, is controversial, but we chose to use it here rather than engage in a dialogue about the most appropriate term.

oped a second innovative program, a dream-sharing group that allowed women to reveal their anxieties and traumas through a culturally congruent approach (Thompson, 1991). In a third program, crocheting, English lessons, and relaxation tapes were the activities highlighted.

Other approaches to tailoring programs to unique populations are choosing hours that fit immigrant women's lifestyle and child care responsibilities, gender matching of clients and providers, providing transportation and child care, giving repeated access to the same caregiver, providing interpreter services, creating community outreach programs, and accommodating or excluding family members in caregiving as requested by clients.

A group of women immigrants may also manifest unique risks and vulnerabilities to particular illnesses or health-compromising situations because of prior life experiences. Providing care utilizing the uniqueness principle also requires using a developmental framework, a staging approach that helps providers consider length of time in the United States, facility with the English language, change in educational level, size of the ethnic community, and changes in living arrangements over the years.

Time

Time is required to develop trust in a program and those who staff it, particularly for women who escaped from situations of war, political oppression, or torture. Nurse encounters with immigrant women require sufficient time for trust to develop to uncover explanatory frameworks of those whose transitions or encounters with xenophobia further marginalize them. Such encounters require mutual understanding. However, while language interpreters may help, they often provide only literal translation because of time limitations. Translations that include nuances and symbolic meanings are often needed.

A culturally competent program for immigrant women allows time for story telling and narrative discourse. Many clients who appear silent in health care encounters are quite verbal when given enough time to express themselves. They are not accustomed to the Euro-American communication style based on short answers to short questions. Instead, they often need to be able to tell a story that illuminates their situation and symptoms without time limitations. If women cannot relate their stories, health care providers may have incomplete information on which to base diagnoses and treatment. Staff in such programs must be able to examine their own values and communication styles and free themselves to respect different values and ways of communicating.

Another time-intensive characteristic is advocacy, a cornerstone of nursing practice essential when caring for clients who need it. A common characteristic of the exemplars is flexibility in termination of services. Women can stay with the program as long as they need or want to. In these exemplars, women who are unsure of what they need can seek help in clarifying and meeting their needs.

Personal, Contextual, and Comprehensive

Common characteristics of the exemplars are their personal orientation, comprehensiveness, and design based on the life context, usual activities, likes, and needs of women (e.g., quilting, sewing, child care, cultural activities, dream telling, peer conversation, and counseling). Common themes in the exemplars are family and community involvement in planning or providing the services. Based on holistic health care principles, these programs recognize the connection between physical and psychological symptoms. Such an approach reaches even "hard to reach" populations. An example is the group of depressed, isolated, middle-aged and elderly women refugees resettled from Cambodia with little or no English-language skills or formal education, and a history of multiple major losses, who were also isolated from the younger generation of their ethnic group. These women manifested unrelenting physical symptoms such as headaches and intractable abdominal pain. The intervention for these women, while clinic-based, consisted of nonclinical gatherings with peers led by a clinician with whom they had developed trust during primary-care clinic visits. It seems highly useful to house culturally competent programs in the neighborhood and to rely on innovative outreach strategies to reach both the hard-to-reach and "invisible" population.

Another common element of the exemplars is the personal nature of services offered. Developing trust and enhancing communication requires time and consistency of staff. Having the same person provide care over time enhances trust, ensures continuity, enhances compliance, and decreases misinterpretation of information. In addition, in these exemplars, personal boundaries between health care providers and clients are blurred. Staff are "people" to clients, rather than being seen only in their clinical roles—sharing their own lives and reciprocating in developing and maintaining relationships. In other words, boundaries between the personal and the clinical vary in different populations, and culturally competent programs are built on understanding these boundaries.

Empowering

Another common principle in the exemplars is their empowering aspects. Participants are given options, valued as individuals, and invited to share their thoughts. Their experiences are considered significant and germane to the issues at hand. Empowerment occurs through participating in decisions, knowing options, being supported and valued, and being in a position to negotiate on an equal basis (Connelly, Keele, Kleinbeck, Schneider, & Cobb, 1993). To empower is to value, to eliminate stereotyping, to decrease isolation and alienation, to develop partnerships, to enhance involvement, to support collectivity, and to provide and support options and choices (Shields, 1995). If we listen to stories, build solidarity, offer protection, and change environments that are marginalizing, we empower clients. When we do that, we can make major contributions to decreasing clients' health risks and enhancing their quality of life. In addition, as we empower our clients we also empowers ourselves.

Policy Recommendations and Proposed Strategies

To make fundamental advances in social justice for women immigrants, essential policy discussions are necessary at several levels. We make nine policy recommendations in this monograph, which are described below and also listed in Appendix B. The first two are national strategies, the next two are public or private, and the last five suggest priorities for nursing organizations.

Proposed National Strategies

A national health program offering universal access regardless of legal status should guarantee the availability of appropriate health care to immigrant women. Instead, in 1994, the U.S. Congress rejected national health insurance and, in 1996, reversed the direction of six decades of social welfare policy. The welfare reform law enacted in 1996 affects more than food stamps and cash assistance to needy families with children. It also affects medical assistance through Medicaid, which has been historically linked to welfare.

The Personal Responsibility and Work Opportunity Reconciliation Act of 1996 contains complex provisions to tighten immigrants' access to cash assistance. These provisions, too, affect access to Medicaid. For example, an immigrant woman coming to the United States in the future would be ineligible for Medicaid for 5 years, except for emergency care. Were she to become pregnant, Medicaid would not be available for prenatal care. For the next 5 years, she may be eligible for Medicaid if, first, her state has chosen to cover "qualified immigrants," and if, second, she meets the definition of "qualified immigrant." But, even in this second 5-year period, her sponsor's income will be "deemed" to be her income along with her own income. If she now becomes pregnant, she will likely fail the means (that is, income and assets) test for Medicaid. Again, she will not have coverage for prenatal care.

Proposals to restore eligibility and benefits cut by the Personal Responsibility and Work Opportunity Reconciliation Act of 1996 must move forward.

Proposed restorations affecting Medicaid coverage, as well as proposals to change Medicare, must consider immigrant women based on careful and adequate analysis of their needs. Thus, the first policy recommendation is:

> *1. Aid to immigrants must be restored and expanded in order to assure that women have timely access to needed health care services regardless of legal status.*

Another pressing public policy issue frequently identified by community advocates, health care planners, health care providers, and researchers is the need for sufficient data on numbers and needs in specific immigrant populations. Inadequate data collection and analysis make it difficult to define problems and nearly impossible to determine the extent of need in immigrant populations. Local communities and providers have attempted to respond to some urgent needs but have little capacity to determine if their programs address root causes. Current social classifications are too limited to extrapolate to the socioeconomic and health status of many immigrant groups. Research and programs that focus on African-American, Hispanic, Asian/Pacific Islander, and Native Americans lump together very different populations and leave out many more. For instance, in communities with large Middle-Eastern immigrant populations, there are no data about the prevalence of infant mortality and low birth weight babies. Local and state public health authorities do not know whether to provide programs for Middle Eastern immigrants in general or for specific groups, such as Palestinians or Chaldeans. Too often in these circumstances, state and local agencies respond to demands of aggressive advocates without adequate support based on data and analysis.

In April 1997, the United States Bureau of the Census recommended to Congress that ancestry data be included in the year 2000 census. Such data are critical to our understanding of what is happening to immigrant populations. Administrative changes for improved definitions and data proposed here will provide minimal benefit without ancestry data from the census. Therefore, the second policy recommendation is:

> *2. Administrative rules and regulations should be developed to broaden the current coding of data collected at federal and state levels to encompass multiple ethnic and racial subgroups.*

Proposed Public and Private Strategies

The overall recommended strategy involves grant making and program implementation in both public and private sectors. In essence, this strategy is to promote "models of excellence," such as the programs described in Appendix A. To bring excellent programs to all our nation's immigrant women, models should be further identified, developed, sustained, expanded, and replicated. Specific strategies are:

> *3. Private foundations, state and local governments, and other state and local organizations should continue to support model development in demonstration projects and their linkages with more comprehensive integrated health delivery systems.*

Energy must be focused on service-delivery models, the development and replication of which are critical to meeting health needs of immigrant women. A key to sustainability can be to link into comprehensive health, social service, and educational systems. Anchoring such programs into larger systems can help their survival while also increasing the cultural appropriateness and cost-effectiveness of the larger systems.

> *4. Private foundations, state and local governments, and other state and local organizations should assist and support the development of self-help and support groups.*

Local mutual aid societies, self-help, and support groups have been effective in helping immigrants cope with new environments. Often these groups have been the primary sources for counseling, referral, and financial support to meet emergencies. These groups have also attempted to initiate mechanisms for monitoring issues and defining the groups' priority needs.

Priorities for Nursing Organizations
We propose five priorities for nursing organizations. The first is a process by which such organizations as Sigma Theta Tau International and the American Academy of Nursing can sustain members' work on immigrant women's health. Two more priorities are proposed partnering activities directed toward policy, research, and education. The remaining two priorities are aimed at defining how nursing organizations can actively participate in implementing one of the recommended policies and one of the strategies.

> *5. Nurses' interest groups concerned with women's health and international health should join forces for concentrated developmental work on knowledge, skill, and action that make such groups successful and recognized champions of immigrant women's health. Many special committees and interest groups on women's health and on international health exist within nurses' organizations.*

This monograph could be the launching pad for a series of forums held yearly in conjunction with, for example, the Academy of Nursing's annual meetings. Joint work by the interest groups should focus on inaugurating the other four priority activities and carrying forward progressively more sophisticated and effective work. Each annual forum could be enriched by the prior year's experience in implementing these activities. The forums could be primary vehicles for shaping participation in the ongoing policy dialogues called for in this working document.

The monograph should also be a launching pad for research. We suggest that members of Sigma Theta Tau International and the Academy of Nursing participate in answering some pressing research questions such as these: What do immigrant women do to keep themselves and other women healthy? What works, what doesn't? What are immigrant women's greatest health and safety concerns for themselves and for other women they know? What do immigrant women understand about their rights as patients and about informed consent? What do immigrant women understand about state and national laws and how the laws affect them? What is taught in basic nursing program curricula about gender and ethical issues in health care, about cultural concepts of health and cross-cultural communication, and about immigrants? What are the patterns of reproductive morbidity among immigrant women?

> 6. *Nursing organizations should work proactively with other organizations to develop a focused policy-informing strategy and a research agenda on women, health, and poverty.*

Although many divisions and turf issues separate the health professions, consensus can be reached in certain areas. For example, important areas are developing public policies, advocating for change, defining issues, identifying human resource needs, increasing resources for national collection of health-status data, and support and direction for research. The exemplars of culturally appropriate health care described here presuppose having nurses with the requisite knowledge and skills to practice with sensitivity to the unique needs of immigrant women and other marginalized populations. To this end, nurse education programs should incorporate content and learning experiences that prepare future nurses for effective work with underserved communities, including immigrant women and their families.

> 7. *Nursing organizations should address how they can work among themselves and with other appropriate groups to ensure that all health professional students are introduced to explicit processes for de-*

*veloping appropriate culturally sensitive interven-
tions and have related learning experiences in clinical and community settings to reinforce the learning.*

*8. Nursing organizations should address how they
might facilitate identification and dissemination of
strategies that work for collecting and analyzing
health-status data at local levels.*

The absence of appropriate health-status data for immigrant groups is a
serious and major gap, particularly in this time of change in which access
to care has been severely compromised. A critical need exists for popula-
tion-specific data that can support policy and program development. The
recommendation from the Census Bureau to Congress on ancestry data is
controversial. Many advocates have temporarily abandoned that recommendation, although a coalition of immigration groups is active concerning the
issue. The public awareness of the "Tiger Woods phenomenon" must not
be allowed to overshadow the importance of recognizing, rather than blur-
ring, distinctions between racial and ethnic groups and subgroups for purposes of measuring health status.

*9. Members of nursing organizations should address
how they might facilitate the identification and dissemination of health and human service models
and programs that work.*

Conclusions

Immigrant women have often been normalized, marginalized, or ignored. Providing care that is culturally competent is a necessity and is also demanded by clients. A nursing perspective requires that we develop culturally competent care by using a framework that recognizes the environment that marginalizes our clients and that seeks to reduce environmental constraints in the health of immigrant women.

Many issues are involved in caring for immigrant women and indications are that their situation is being recognized by lawmakers. An example is this excerpt from *The Earth Times*:

> The U.S. Immigration and Naturalization Service (INS) just issued new guidelines that take into account specific types of persecution suffered by women only. Rape, domestic abuse, infanticide, genital mutilation, slavery, forced abortion, and forced marriages are examples of gender-based discrimination that may provide reasons to grant asylum. But claimants will have to show how their political beliefs are at odds with those in power, and as a result of those differences how they face persecution sanctioned by their governments. Recently, the INS granted asylum to a Haitian woman [because she was] a victim of gang-rape. Government soldiers [had] attacked her because she supported then-exiled President Jean-Bertrand Aristide. In another case, a Jordanian woman received asylum because her husband beat her and the government refused to help her, in effect, sanctioning his behavior" (pp. 15-29: June 1995).

The four purposes set forth for this working document were, in summary, to (a) frame the issues and risks for immigrant women's health, (b) identify programmatic models of excellence, (c) analyze principles for culturally competent care, and (d) make recommendations related to access, quality, wellness, and safety.

A need exists for ongoing policy dialogues. These ongoing policy dialogues should be set in the wider context of policy redirection to implement principles of social justice for all disenfranchised groups. As is true for other populations at risk, immigrant women will be best served by policies that encourage and facilitate pursuit of individual freedom and that provide universal access to economic opportunity and income security, education and training, appropriate health care, affordable housing, and safe communities. This "olive paper" supports the need for mechanisms for collecting better data on health status; research agendas to define essential issues and develop and test models of intervention; educational programs to improve health care providers' knowledge and skills to better care for immigrant women; and strategic advocacy by professional, civic, and community organizations.

SECTION

VII.

References

Amnesty International. (1995). **Women in Afghanistan: A human rights catastrophe**. New York: Amnesty International, USA.

Anderson, J.M. (1987). Migration and health: Perspectives on immigrant women. **Sociology of Health & Illness, 9**, 410-438.

Anderson, J.M. (1991). Immigrant women speak of chronic illness: The social construction of the devalued self. **Journal of Advanced Nursing, 16**, 710-717.

Antonovsky, A. (1979). **Health, stress and coping**. San Francisco, CA: Jossey-Bass.

Aroian, K.J. (1990). A model of psychological adaptation to migration and resettlement. **Nursing Research, 39**, 5-10.

Barbee, E.L. (1987). Tensions in the brokerage role: Nurses in Botswana. **Western Journal of Nursing Research, 9**, 244-256.

Bechtel, G.A., Shepherd, M.A., & Rogers, P.W. (1995). Family, culture, and health practices among migrant farmworkers. **Journal of Community Health Nursing, 12**, 15-22.

Boyd, M. (1984). At a disadvantage: The occupational attainments of foreign born women in Canada. **International Migration Review, 18**, 1091-1119.

Budman, C.L., Lipson, J.G., & Meleis, A.I. (1992). The cultural consultant in mental health care. **American Journal of Orthopsychiatry, 62**, 359-370.

Castro, F., Baezconde-Garbanati, L., & Beltran, H. (1985). Risk factors for coronary heart disease in Hispanic populations: A review. **Hispanic Journal of Behavioral Science, 7**, 153-175.

Chick, N., & Meleis, A.I. (1986). Transitions: A nursing concern. In P.L. Chinn (Ed.), **Nursing research methodology** (pp. 237-257). Boulder, CO: Aspen Publications.

Cobas, J., Balcazar, H., Benin, M., Keith, V., & Chong, Y. (1996). Acculturation and low-birth weight infants among Latino [sic] women: A reanalysis of HHANES data with structural equation models. **American Journal of Public Health, 86**, 394-396.

Connelly, L.M., Keele, B.S., Kleinbeck, S.V.M., Schneider, J.K., & Cobb, A.K. (1993). A place to be yourself: Empowerment from the client's perspective. **Image: Journal of Nursing Scholarship, 25**, 297-303.

El Sayed, Y.A. (1986). **The successive-unsettled transitions of migration and their impact on postpartum concerns of Arab immigrant women**. Unpublished doctoral dissertation, University of California, San Francisco.

Faludi, S. (1991). **Backlash**. New York, NY: Crown Publishers.

Flaskerud, J.H. (1987). A proposed protocol for culturally relevant nursing psychotherapy. **Clinical Nurse Specialist, 1**, 150-157.

Flavell, C. (1994). Women and coronary heart disease. **Progress in Cardiovascular Nursing, 9(4)**, 18-27.

Franks, F., & Faux, S.A. (1990). Depression, stress, mastery, and social resources in four ethnocultural women's groups. **Research in Nursing & Health, 13**, 283-292.

Gilligan, C. (1982). **In a different voice**. Cambridge, MA: Harvard University Press.

Hahn, R., & Muecke, M. (1987). Ethnic variation in birth outcomes. Implications for obstetrical practice. **Current Problems in Obstetrics, Gynecology and Fertility, 10**, 133-171.

Hall, J.A., Stevens, P.E., & Meleis, A.I. (1994). Marginalization: A guiding concept for valuing diversity in nursing knowledge development. **Advances in Nursing Science, 16**, 23-41.

Hattar-Pollara, M., & Meleis, A.I. (1995a). Stress of immigration and the daily lived experiences of Jordanian immigrant women in the United States. **Western Journal of Nursing Research, 17**, 521-538.

Hattar-Pollara, M., & Meleis, A.I. (1995b). Parenting their adolescents: The experiences of Jordanian immigrant women in California. **Health Care for Women International, 16**, 195-211.

Heiss, L., Patting, J., & Germaine, A. (1994). **Violence against women: The hidden health burden**. Washington, DC: The World Bank.

Jezewski, M.A. (1990). Culture brokering in migrant farmworkers health care. **Western Journal of Nursing Research, 12**, 497-513.

Juarbe, T. (1996). The state of Hispanic health: Cardiovascular disease and health. In S. Torres (Ed.), **Hispanic voices: Hispanic health educators speak out** (pp. 93-113). NY: National League of Nursing.

Jones, J.F. (1988). Southeast Asian refugees, mental health, and professional training. **Social Development Issues, 12**, 42-47.

Kagan, A., Harris, B., Winkelstein, W., Johnson, K., Kato, H., Hamilton, H., Syme, S., Rhoads, G., Gay, M., & Nichaman, M. (1974). Epidemiological studies of coronary heart disease and stroke in Japanese men living in Japan, Hawaii, and California: Demographic, physical, dietary, and biochemical characteristics. **Journal of Chronic Disease, 27**, 345-364.

Kleinman, A. (1980). **Patients and healers in the context of culture**. Berkeley, CA: University of California Press.

Kulig, J.C. (1990). A review of the health status of Southeast Asian refugee women. **Health Care for Women International, 11**, 49-63.

Lalonde, R.N., Taylor, D.M., & Moghaddam, F.M. (1992). The process of social identification for visible immigrant women in a multicultural context. **Journal of Cross-Cultural Psychology, 23**, 25-39.

Lipson, J.G. (1992). Iranian immigrants: Health and adjustment. **Western Journal of Nursing Research, 14**, 10-29.

Lipson, J.G., & Miller, S. (1994). Changing roles of Afghan refugee women in the U.S. **Health Care for Women International, 15**, 171-180.

Lipson, J.G., Hosseini, T., Kabir, S., Omidian, P., & Edmonston, F. (1995). Health Issues Among Afghan Women in California. **Health Care for Women International, 16**, 279-286.

Lipson, J.G., & Omidian, P. (1997). Afghan refugee issues in the U.S. social environment. **Western Journal of Nursing Research, 19**, 110-126.

Magnusson, G., & Aurelius, G. (1980). Illness behavior and nationality: A study of hospital care utilization by immigrants and natives in a Stockholm district. **Social Science and Medicine, 14A**, 357-362.

Mahon, J., McFarlane, J., & Golden, K. (1991). De madres a madres: A community partnership for health. **Public Health Nursing, 8**, 15-19.

Meleis, A.I. (1991). Between two cultures: Identity, roles, and health. **Health Care for Women International, 12**, 365-354.

Meleis, A.I., & Bernal, P. (1996). The paradoxical world daily domestic workers in Cali, Colombia. **Human Organization, 55**, 393-400.

Meleis, A.I., Norbeck, J.S., Laffrey, S.C., Solomon, M., & Miller, L. (1989). Stress, satisfaction, and coping: A study of women clerical workers. **Health Care for Women International, 8**, 319-334.

Meleis, A.I., Isenberg, M., Koerner, J., & Stern, P. (1995). **Diversity, marginalization, and culturally-competent health care: Issues in knowledge development**. Washington, DC: American Academy of Nursing.

Meleis, A.I., Douglas, M., Eribes, C., Shih, F., & Messias, D. (1996). Employed Mexican women as mothers and partners: Valued, empowered and overloaded. **Journal of Advanced Nursing, 23**, 82-90.

Meleis, A.I. (1995). Immigrant women in borderless societies: Marginalized and empowered. **Asian Journal of Nursing Studies**, October, 39-47.

Mirdal, G.M. (1984). Stress and distress in migration: Problems and resources of Turkish women in Denmark. **International Migration Review, 18**, 984-1003.

Mendoza, F., Ventura, S., Burciaga-Valdez, R., Castillo, R., Escoto Saldiva, L., Baisden, K., & Martorell, R. (1991). Selected measures of health status for Mexican-American, Puerto Rican, and Cuban-American children. **JAMA, 265**, 227-232.

Muecke, M. (1987). Resettled refugees' reconstruction of identity: Lao in Seattle. **Urban Anthropology and Studies of Cultural Systems and World Economic Development, 16**, 273-289.

Muecke, M. (1992). New paradigms for refugee health problems. **Social Science and Medicine, 35**, 515-523.

National Council for Research on Women. (1995). The Lucy Parsons' initiative: Laying the groundwork for contingent women workers. **Issues Quarterly, 1(3)**, 22-23.

Nelson, M. (1995). **Role involvement, availability of resources and health practices among low-income working women**. Unpublished doctoral dissertation, University of California, San Francisco.

Ogur, B. (1990). Mental health problems of translocated women. **Health Care for Women International, 11**, 43-47

Omidian, P., & Lipson, J. (1996). Ethnic coalitions and public health: Delights and dilemmas in the Afghan Health Education Project. **Human Organization, 55**, 355-360.

Pessar, P.R. (1984). The linkage between the household and workplace of Dominican women in the United States. **International Migration Review, 18**, 1188-1211.

Rankin, S. (1989). Women recovering from cardiac surgery [Abstract]. **Circulation, 80** (Suppl.), II-391.

Rumbaut, R. (1985). Mental health and the refugee experience; A comparative study of Southeast Asian refugees. In T.C. Owan (Ed.), **Southeast Asian mental health, treatment, prevention, services, training and research**, (pp. 433-486). Rockville, MD: National Institutes of Mental Health.

Sanders-Phillips, K. (1994). Health promotion behavior in low income Black and Latino women. **Women & Health, 21**, 71-83.

Schumacher, K., & Meleis, A.I. (1994). Transitions: A central concept in nursing. **Image: Journal of Nursing Scholarship, 26**, 119-127.

Scribner, R., & Dwyer, J. (1989). Acculturation and low birth weight among Latinos in the Hispanic HANES. **American Journal of Public Health, 79**, 1263-1267.

Shields, L. (1995). Women's experiences of the meaning of empowerment. **Qualitative Health Research, 5**, 15-35.

Stevens, P.E., Hall, J.M., & Meleis, A.I. (1992). Examining vulnerability of women clerical workers from five ethnic/racial groups. **Western Journal of Nursing Research, 14**, 754-774.

Stier, H. (1991). Immigrant women go to work: Analysis of immigrant wives' labor supply for six Asian groups. **Social Science Quarterly, 72**, 67-82.

The Earth Times (1995, June). (pp. 15-29).

Thompson, J.L. (1991). Exploring gender and culture with Khmer refugee women: Reflections on participatory feminist research. **Advances in Nursing Science, 13**, 30-48.

Tienda, M., Jensen, L., & Bach, R.L. (1984). Immigration, gender and the process of occupational change in the United States, 1970-80. **International Migration Review, 18**, 1021-1044.

Tripp-Reimer, T., & Brink, P. (1984). Culture brokerage. In Bulechek & McCloskey (Eds.), **Nursing interventions** (pp. 352-364). New York: W.B. Saunders.

Van der Stuyft, P., De Muynck, A., Schillemans, L., & Timmerman, C. (1989). Migration, acculturation and utilization of primary health care. **Social Science and Medicine, 29**, 53-60.

Vega, W.A., Kolody, B., Valle, R., & Weir, J. (1991). Social networks, social support, and their relationship to depression among immigrant Mexican women. **Human Organization, 50**, 154-162.

Vega, W.A., Kolody, B., & Valle, R. (1987). Migration and mental health: An empirical test of depression risk factors among immigrant Mexican women. **International Migration Review, 21**, 512-530.

Vega, W.A., Kolody, B., Valle, R., & Hough, R. (1986). Depressive symptoms and their correlates among immigrant Mexican women in the United States. **Social Science and Medicine, 22**, 645-652.

Ying, Y.W. (1990). Explanatory models of major depression and implications for help-seeking among immigrant Chinese-American women. **Culture, Medicine and Psychiatry, 14**, 393-408.

SECTION VIII.

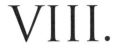

Bibliography

WOMEN'S ROLES: GENDER, FAMILY, AND WORK

Amott, T., & Matthaei, J. (1991). Climbing gold Mountain: Asian American Women. In **Race, gender, and work** (pp. 193-256). Boston, MA: South End Press.

Boyd, M. (1991). Immigration and living arrangements: Elderly women in Canada. **International Migration Review, 25(1)**, 4-27.

Chamnivickorn, S. (1988). Fertility, labor supply and investment in child quality among Asian American immigrant women. **Pacific Asian American Mental Health Research Review, 6**, 28-29.

Dallalfar, A. (1994). Iranian women as immigrant entrepreneurs. **Gender and Society, 8**, 541-561.

Fox, P. G., Cowell, J.M., & Johnson, M. (1995). The effects of family disruption on Southeast Asian refugee women: Implications for international nursing. **International Nursing Review, 42**, 27-30.

Keefe, S.E., Padilla, A.M., & Carlos, M.L. (1979). The Mexican-American extended family as an emotional support system. **Human Organization, 38**, 145-152.

Kelly, G.P. (1994). To become an American woman: Education and sex role socialization of the Vietnamese immigrant woman. In V.L. Ruiz & E.C. DuBois (Eds.), **Unequal Sisters: A multicultural reader in U.S. women's history** (pp. 497-507). New York: Routledge.

Krulfeld, R.M. (1994). Buddhism, maintenance and change: Reinterpreting gender in a Lao refugee community. In L. Camino & R. Krulfeld (Eds.), **Reconstructing lives, recapturing meaning** (pp. 97-127). Basel: Gordon and Breach.

Kulig, J. (1994). Old traditions in a new world: Changing gender relations among Cambodian refugees. In L. Camino & R. Krulfeld (Eds.), **Reconstructing lives, recapturing meaning** (pp.129-146). Basel: Gordon and Breach.

Lipson, J.G., & Miller, S. (1994). Changing roles of Afghan women in the United States. **Health Care for Women International, 15**, 171-180.

Meleis, A.I. (1990). Between two cultures: Identity, roles, and health. **Health Care for Women International, 12**, 365-377.

Meleis, A.I., & Rogers, S. (1987). Women in transition: Being versus becoming or being and becoming. **Health Care for Women International, 8**, 199-217.

Muecke, M. (1995). Trust, abuse of trust, and mistrust among refugee women from Cambodia: A cultural interpretation. In J. C. Knudsen & E. V. Daniel (Eds.), **Mistrusting Refugees** (pp. 36-55). Berkeley: University of California Press.

National Council for Research on Women. (1995). The Lucy Parsons' initiative: Laying the groundwork for contingent women workers. **Issues Quarterly, 1(3)**, 22-23.

Parvanta, S. (1992). The balancing act: Plight of Afghan women refugees: The challenges and rewards. In E. Cole, O. Espin, & E. Rothblum (Eds.), **Refugee women and their mental health: Shattered societies, shattered lives** (pp. 113-128). New York: Haworth Press.

Repak, T.A. (1994). Labor recruitment and the lure of the capital: Central American migrants in Washington, DC. **Gender & Society, 8**, 507-524.

Thompson, J.L. (1991). Exploring gender and culture with Khmer refugee women: Reflections on participatory feminist research. **Advances in Nursing Science, 13(3)**, 30-48.

Weitzman, B.C., & Berry, C.A. (1992). Health status and health care utilization among New York City home attendants: An illustration of needs of working poor, immigrant women. **Women and Health, 19**, 87-105.

Yee, B.W.K. (1992). Markers of successful aging among Vietnamese refugee women. In E. Cole, O. Espin, & E. Rothblum (Eds.), **Refugee women and their mental health: Shattered societies, shattered lives** (pp. 221-238). New York: Haworth Press.

Zsembik, B.A., & Peek, C.W. (1994). The effect of economic restructuring on Puerto Rican women's labor force participation in the formal sector. **Gender & Society, 8**, 525-540.

HEALTH CARE ISSUES
Sources/Areas of Vulnerability

Anderson, J. (1991). Immigrant women speak of chronic illness: The social construction of the devalued self. **Journal of Advanced Nursing, 16**, 710-717.

Calhoun, M. (1985). The Vietnamese woman: Health/illness attitudes and behaviors. **Health Care for Women International, 6**, 61-72.

Canadian Task Force on Mental Health Issues Affecting Immigrants and Refugees. (1988). In **Belser et al., After the door has been opened**. Health and Welfare Canada.

Cole, E., Espin, O., & Rothblum, E. (Eds.). (1992). **Refugee women and their mental health: Shattered societies, shattered lives**. New York: Haworth Press.

Franks, F., & Faux, S. (1990). Depression, stress, mastery and social resources in four ethnocultural women's groups. **Research in Nursing and Health, 13**, 283-292.

Fruchter, R.G., Remy, J.C., Boyce, J.G., & Burnett, W.S. (1986). Cervical cancer in immigrant women. **American Journal of Public Health, 76**, 797-799.

Herbst, P.K.R. (1992). From helpless victim to empowered survivor: Oral history as a treatment for survivors of torture. In E. Cole, O. Espin, & E. Rothblum (Eds.), **Refugee women and their mental health: Shattered societies, shattered lives** (pp.141-154). New York: Haworth Press.

Juarbe, T. (1994). **Factors that influence diet and exercise experiences of immigrant Mexican women**. Unpublished dissertation, University of California, San Francisco.

Kulig, J. (1988). Conception and birth control use: Cambodian refugee women's beliefs and practices. **Journal of Community Health Nursing, 5**, 235-246.

Kulig, J. (1990). Childbearing beliefs among Cambodian refugee women. **Western Journal of Nursing Research, 12**, 108-118.

Kulig, J. (1990). A review of the health status of Southeast Asian refugee women. **Health Care for Women International, 11**, 49-63.

Lipson, J.G. (1993). Afghan refugees in California: Mental health issues. **Issues in Mental Health Nursing, 14**, 411-423.

Lipson, J.G., Hosseini, T., Kabir, S., Omidian, P., & Edmonston, F. (1995). Health issues among Afghan women in California. **Health Care for Women International, 16**, 279-286.

Muecke, M., & Hahn, R. (1987). Ethnic variation in birth outcomes: Implications for obstetrical practice. **Current Problems in Obstetrics, Gynecology and Fertility, 10**, 133-171.

Muecke, M.A., & Sassi, L. (1992). Anxiety among Cambodian refugee adolescents in transit and in resettlement. **Western Journal of Nursing Research, 14**, 267-285.

Muecke, M.A. (1992). New paradigms for refugee health problems. **Social Science and Medicine, 35**, 515-523.

Pang, K.Y.C. (1990). Hwabyung: The construction of a Korean popular illness among Korean elderly immigrant women in the United States. **Culture, Medicine and Psychiatry, 14**, 495-512.

Saldaña, D.H. (1992). **Coping with stress: A refugee's story**. In E. Cole, O. Espin, & E. Rothblum (Eds.), **Refugee women and their mental health: Shattered societies, shattered lives** (pp. 21-33). New York: Haworth Press.

Shepard, J., & Faust, S. (1993). Refugee health care and the problem of suffering. **Bioethics Forum, 9(3)**, 3-7.

Shin, K.R. (1993). Factors predicting depression among Korean-American women in New York. **International Journal of Nursing Studies, 30**, 415-423.

Vega, W.A., Kolody, B., Valle, R., & Weir, J. (1991). Social networks, social support, and their relationship to depression among immigrant Mexican women. **Social Science and Medicine, 50**, 154-162.

Vega, W.A., Kolody, B. & Valle, J. (1987). Migration and mental health: An empirical test of depression risk factors among immigrant Mexican women. **International Migration Review, 21**, 512-529.

U.S. Department of Health & Human Services. (1992, June 5). Prevention and control of tuberculosis in migrant farm workers. Recommendations of the Advisory Council for the elimination of Tuberculosis. **MMWR, 41**, RR-10. PHS, CDC, Atlanta.

U.S. Department of Health & Human Services. (1990, Dec. 28). Tuberculosis among foreign-born persons entering the United States: Recommendations of the Advisory Council for the Elimination of Tuberculosis. **MMWR, 39**, RR-18, 28. Atlanta.

BARRIERS/CONCERNING ACCESS TO CARE

DeSantis, L., & Thomas, J. (1992). Health education and the immigrant Haitian mother: Cultural insights for community health nurses. **Public Health Nursing, 9**, 87-96.

Faller, H. (1985). Perinatal needs of immigrant Hmong women: Surveys of women and health care providers. **Public Health Reports, 100**, 340-343.

Hatton, D.C. (1992). Information transmission in bilingual, bicultural contexts. **Journal of Community Health Nursing, 9**, 53-59.

Hatton, D., & Webb, T. (1993). Information transmission in bilingual, bicultural contexts: A field study of community health nurses and interpreters. **Journal of Community Health, 10**, 137-147.

Juarbe, T. (1995). Access to health care for Hispanic women: A primary health care perspective. **Nursing Outlook, 43**, 23-28.

Lipson, J.G., & Meleis, A.I. (1983). Issues in health care of Middle Eastern patients. **Western Journal of Medicine, 139**, 854-861.

Lipson, J.G., & Meleis, A.I. (1985). Culturally appropriate care: The case of immigrants. **Topics in Clinical Nursing, 7**, 48-56.

Luna, L. (1994). Care and cultural context of Lebanese Muslim immigrants: Using Leininger's theory. **Journal of Transcultural Nursing, 5**, 12-20.

Macintyre, M., & Dennerstein, L. (1995). **Shifting latitudes, changing attitudes: Immigrant women's health experiences, attitudes, knowledge and beliefs.** Melbourne, Australia: Key Centre for Women's Health in Society.

Magar, V. (1990). Health care needs of Central American refugees. **Nursing Outlook, 38**, 239-342.

Mattson, S., & Lew, L. (1992). Culturally sensitive prenatal care for Southeast Asians. **Journal of Obstetric, Gynecologic, and Neonatal Nursing, 21**, 48-54.

Minkler, D. (1983). The role of a community-based satellite clinic in the perinatal care of non-English speaking immigrants. **The Western Journal of Medicine, 139**, 905-909.

Muecke, M. (1983). In search of healing: Southeast Asian refugees in the American health care system. **Western Journal of Medicine, 139**, 835-840.

Ong, A. (1995). Making the biopolitical subject: Cambodian immigrants, refugee medicine and cultural citizenship. **Social Science & Medicine, 40**, 1243-1257.

Weitzman, B.C., & Berry, C.A. (1992). Health status and health care utilization among New York City home attendants: An illustration of needs of working poor, immigrant women. **Women and Health, 19**, 87-105.

HEALTH AND ILLNESS RESPONSES

Anderson, J.M. (1985). Perspectives on the health of immigrant women: A feminist analysis. **Advances in Nursing Science, 8**, 61-76.

Calloway, H. (1987). Refugee women: Specific requirements and untapped resources. In G. Altaf (Ed.), **Third world affairs** (pp. 320-325). London: Third World Affairs Foundation.

Frye, B.A., & D'Avanzo, C.D. (1994). Themes in managing culturally defined illness in the Cambodian refugee family. **Journal of Community Health Nursing, 11**, 89-98.

Meleis, A.I., Omidian, P.A., & Lipson, J.G. (1993). Women's health status in the United States: An immigrant women's project. In B. J. McElmurry (Ed.), **Women's Health and development: A global challenge** (pp. 163-181). Boston: Jones & Bartlett.

IMMIGRATION TRANSITION, PROCESS, ADJUSTMENT

Boone, M.S. (1994). Thirty-year retrospective on the adjustment of Cuban refugee women. In L. Camino & R. Krulfeld (Eds.), **Reconstructing lives, recapturing meaning** (pp.179-201). Basel: Gordon and Breach.

Buijs, G. (1993). **Migrant women: Crossing boundaries and changing identities**. Oxford: Berg.

Centre for Documentation on Refugees (CDR). (1989). Refugee women: Selected and annotated bibliography. Geneva: United Nations High Commissioner for Refugees.

DeVoe, P.A. (1992). The silent majority: Women as refugees. In R. Gallin, A. Ferguson, & J. Harper (Eds.), **The women and international development annual, 3** (pp. 19-49). Boulder, CO: Westview Press.

Hongdagneu-Sotelo, P. (1994). **Gendered transitions: Mexican experiences of immigration**. Berkeley: University of California Press.

Martin, S.F. (1991). **Refugee Women**. London and New Jersey: Zen Books Ltd.

Mayotte, J. (1992). **Refugee Women**. In J. Mayotte (Ed.), Disposable people? The plight of refugees. New York: Orbis Books.

Meleis, A.I., & Rogers, S. (1987). Women in transition: Being versus becoming or being and becoming. **Health Care for Women International, 8**, 199-217.

Muecke, M. (1987). Resettled refugees' reconstruction of identity: Lao in Seattle. **Urban Anthropology and Studies of Cultural Systems and World Economic Development, 16**, 273-289.

Muecke, M., & Sassi, L. (1992). Anxiety among Cambodian refugee adolescents in transit and in resettlement. **Western Journal of Nursing Research, 14**, 267-285.

National Council for Research On Women. (1995). The feminization of immigration. **Issues Quarterly, 1**, 1-7.

Robertson, M.K. (1992). Birth, transformation, and death of refugee identity: Women and girls of the intifada. In E. Cole, O. Aspen, & E. Rothblum (Eds.), **Refugee women and their mental health** (pp. 35-52). New York: Haworth Press.

Rosenthal, D.A., & Feldman, S. S. (1990). The acculturation of Chinese immigrants: Perceived effects on family functioning of length of residence in two cultural contexts. **Journal of Genetic Psychology, 151**, 495-514.

Saldaña, D.H. (1992). Coping with stress: A refugee's story. **In Refugee women and their mental health: Shattered societies, shattered lives** (pp. 21-33). New York: Haworth Press.

Siegel, R.J. (1992). Fifty years later: Am I still an immigrant? In E. Cole, O. Aspen, & E. Rothblum (Eds.), **Refugee women and their mental health** (pp. 105-111). New York: Haworth Press.

Summerfield, H. (1993). Patterns of adaptation: Somali and Bangladeshi women in Britain. **Cross Cultural Perspectives on Women, 7**, 83-98.

Sutton, C. (1992).Some thoughts on gendering and internationalizing out thinking about transnational migrations. In N. Schiller, L. Basch, & C. Blanc-Szanton (Eds.), **Towards a transnational perspective on migration: race, class, ethnicity and nationalism reconsidered** (pp. 241-249). New York: New York Academy of Sciences.

VIOLENCE, TORTURE, HUMAN RIGHTS

Fox, P.G., Cowell, J., & Montgomery, A. (1994). The effects of violence on health and adjustment of Southeast Asian refugee children: An integrative review. **Public Health Nursing, 11**, 195-201.

Fox, P.G., Cowell, J.M., & Montgomery, A. (In press). Premigration violence experience of Southeast Asian refugee children in the United States. **International Journal of Psychiatric Nursing Research**.

Frye, B.A., & D'Avanzo, C.D. (1994). Cultural themes in family stress and violence among Cambodian refugee women in the inner city. **Advances in Nursing Science, 16**, 64-77.

Herbst, P.K.R. (1992). From helpless victim to empowered survivor: Oral history as a treatment for survivors of torture. In E. Cole, O. Aspen, & E. Rothblum (Eds.), **Refugee women and their mental health: Shattered societies, shattered lives** (pp. 141-154). New York: Haworth Press.

Indra, D.M. (1989). Ethnic human rights and feminist theory: Gender implications for refugee studies and practice. **Journal of Refugee Studies, 2**, 221-242.

National Council for Research on Women. (1995). Intervening: Immigrant women and domestic violence. **Issues Quarterly, 1**, 12-13.

RESEARCH METHODS, LITERATURE REVIEWS

Center for Documentation on Refugees. (1989). **Refugee women: Selected and annotated bibliography**. Geneva: Office of the United Nations High Commissioner for Refugees.

DeSantis, L. (1990). Fieldwork with undocumented aliens and other populations at risk. **Western Journal of Nursing Research, 12**, 359-372.

Lynam, M., & Anderson, J. (1986). Generating knowledge for nursing practice: Methodological issues in studying immigrant women. In P. Chinn (Ed.), **Nursing research methodology: Issues and implementation** (pp. 259-274), Rockville, MD: Aspen.

Muecke, M. (1992). Nursing research with refugees: A guide and review. **Western Journal of Nursing Research, 14**, 703-720.

Sawyer, L., Regev, H., Proctor, S., Nelson, M., Messias, D., Barnes, D., & Meleis, A.I. (1995). Matching versus cultural competence in research: Methodological considerations. **Research in Nursing and Health, 18**, 557-567.

Thompson, J.L. (1991). Exploring gender and culture with Khmer refugee women: Reflections on participatory feminist research. **Advances in Nursing Science, 13**, 30-48.

Urrutia-Rojas, X., & Aday, L.A. (1991). A framework for community assessment: Designing and conducting a survey in a Hispanic immigrant and refugee community. **Public Health Nursing, 8**, 20-26.

APPENDIX

A

Culturally Appropriate Programs for Immigrant Women: Exemplars

Program 1:   **Health or Social Service Agency Program**
Cambodian Women's Support Group, San Francisco General Hospital, San Francisco, Calif.

The Refugee Clinic at San Francisco General Hospital serves refugees from all over the world. About 25% of the primary care clinic patients are Cambodians—former rice farmers—illiterate in their own language, who now live in San Francisco's Tenderloin district. They witnessed the Pol Pot massacre and holocaust; many will suffer for the rest of their lives from the torture they experienced and resulting post-traumatic stress disorder (PTSD). Regardless of treatment such as symptomatic therapies, psychotherapy, antidepressants, acupuncture, or traditional healing methods—patients suffering from PTSD return again and again complaining of symptoms such as headaches, abdominal pain, and dizziness.

Cambodian Women's Program
To address PTSD in a more effective way, Shotsy Faust, RN, FNP, and Judith Shepard, DSW, developed a support group program for Cambodian women in their late 30s to mid-60s. All had somatic complaints, none had responded to other therapies, and none had learned English. They all had child-care responsibilities, and many were socially isolated single heads of household. The group did not focus on insight or ask women to share their traumas; this western concept would be intrusive for Cambodian women who believe in fate and Karma and feel grateful to survive and go on with life. Instead, the group focused on psychological strengths—they are survivors—helping them get to know each other and to increase their concentration so they could enter American society through their own community.

Women ($N = 10$-20) attended weekly group meetings lasting about 2 hours. Cookies or oranges were provided and if there was a special event, women brought other foods. The group was facilitated by Dr. Shepard and a Cambodian health worker who understands the language and culture of the patients.

Three components are English as a second language (ESL), crafts, and stress-reduction training. The women learned English with others at their same language level, using games and songs. Post-traumatic stress disorder interferes with concentration, so crocheting was encouraged to build concentration. At first, some women were unable to concentrate long enough to finish any task—even two or three crochet stitches. The group members are now very proud of their completed crafts and hope to sell them.

Relaxation and stress reduction are taught using an audiotape and guided visualization. Many of the women who had severe anxiety, awoke early, had sleep disorders, and had nightmares—now fall asleep as soon as the tape begins. Each woman has her own tape to play at home for help with sleep problems.

Two other concerns emerged from this group—unresolved grief and children's needs. Because the women had been unable to honor family members who had died, Buddhist monks were hired to do group ceremonies to honor dead loved ones—a very healing event. To take care of the children for whom immigrant or refugee women were responsible, a child development worker was hired. And because PTSD has a ripple effect throughout the family, the worker evaluated the children through play therapy at the same time that she provided child care.

The number of clinic visits made by these women have been reduced by 50% and they have fewer complaints. The difference in the women is remarkable; they smile, have a more positive affect, and try to speak English. Suffering has been relieved, which was the goal for the women, and the program was cost-effective, which was the organization's goal.

Abstracted from Refugee Health Care: Problems and Solutions by Shotsy Faust and Juliene Lipson, a paper presented at the annual meeting of the American Anthropological Association, December 3, 1992, San Francisco, Calif.

Reference

Shepard, J., & Faust, S. (1993). Refugee Health Care and the Problem of Suffering. **Bioethics Forum, 9**, 3-7.

Program 2:   Health or Social Service Agency Program
Por La Vida, San Diego, Calif.

Sponsored by a partnership between San Diego State University and the Logan Heights family health center, the Por la Vida program uses a grassroots approach to health promotion in the Latino/Hispanic community. The design and materials are culturally congruent for the Mexican-American community.

The model was originally developed in 1986 with funding from the Kaiser Foundation. The original focus was cardiovascular risk reduction, and it was implemented in San Diego's Latino community with funding from the

Chronic Disease Prevention branch of the California Department of Health Services. In 1989, the project expanded into tobacco prevention, and in 1990, a grant from the National Cancer Institute funded development and implementation of a program on breast and cervical cancer.

The health promotion content and materials were developed by a team of health educators, a dietician, a physician, the Latino community coordinator, and an instructional designer using extensive and on-going community feedback. This ongoing discussion resulted in a list of topics for each series that included both standard health education topics and those that community women felt were very important. For example, in each series, women's self-esteem and available community resources were emphasized.

Implementation of the project began with identification of interested women in the community who had good sized social networks. They were trained using a support group format. Each woman invited a group of her friends and family members to her home for a weekly session on a chosen topic. Information was presented, women discussed it and engaged in activities to reinforce the information. Behavioral changes were assessed on worksheets with individual goal setting designed for low literacy levels.

The cardiovascular disease program included 16 sessions about self-esteem, community resources, exercise, diet, and a supermarket tour. Community living skills included developing positive characteristics, being prepared for earthquakes, personal self-defense, job/vocational training, low cost family activities, budgeting, saving money, parenting skills, amnesty/immigration/citizenship information, and being aware of drug problems. The tobacco abuse prevention program was six sessions focusing on cessation and prevention among women and their families and friends and ended with community action recognizing the tobacco industry's marketing in the Latino community. The cancer prevention curriculum is 12 sessions, including topics about self-esteem, women's anatomy, breast self-examination, pap tests, mammograms, diet, and smoking cessation. Examples of topics for sessions were *fuente*—women's bodies (heart, lungs, genitourinary system), finding out about cancer, keeping the uterus and cervix healthy, keeping breasts healthy, overcoming barriers to pap smears or mammograms, eating well, protecting health, communicating with a daughter or friend, and the dangers of smoking.

The program strengths are implementation in someone's home, in the language chosen by the women, with content at a level appropriate to their needs, in a group who already know each other. Topics are those that the women consider important as well as those health educators consider important. The support-group format helps the women meet their personal goals.

Abstracted from the Por La Vida brochure and materials from the California State Department of Health, Health Promotion Section.

Program 3:   Health or Social Service Agency Program
Mobile Refugee Clinic and Language Bank, Seattle, Wash.

Since 1979, Seattle has become a destination city for refugees coming to the United States from Southeast Asia. Numerous nongovernmental resettlement agencies found the city attractive for its moderate climate, openness to newcomers, and moderate size. The city-county health department quickly responded by setting up a mobile refugee clinic that provided physical screening, immunizations, and referrals to local resources, primarily to community clinics. The Clinic was located in selected communities where refugees and immigrants had been resettled. Health department policy was set early to assure dispersed, rather than centralized, service, in order to meet the new arrivals in their own locations and to support a sense of neighborhood among them and also to use public resources to complement private sector resources and activities.

A cross-sector community ethic of responsibility developed, as evidenced in the emergence of a city-county refugee forum, where service providers, policy makers, and representatives of the various refugee ethnic groups met on a monthly basis to anticipate problems, identify needs, and inform each other of refugee-related developments at city, state, national, and international levels. Also attesting to the community responsibility ethic was the early development of a language bank designed specifically for an interface between non-English speaking patients and English-speaking health care providers. Eventually, the language bank was supported with national grant funds and community resources, as well as by community colleges that developed training programs for interpreters.

The need for trained interpreters was great; requests for interpreters came from the health department, community clinics, hospitals, welfare workers, and even the police and public defenders. As the language-bank program matured, curricula, standards of practice, and evaluation mechanisms were developed; it had a growing reputation for excellence. However, lack of finances became a major barrier to sustaining the program. Grants and government support covered training, health department services, and community clinic services, but no compensation was provided for interpreters' work in hospitals. To meet the mounting fiscal crisis, a "pro bono publicum" group, Evergreen Legal Services, undertook a class-action suit against hospitals. This suit was settled out of court and established a precedent that has subsequently been cited in other situations across the nation. The precedent was that, based upon the 10th amendment to the 1964 Civil Rights Act, federal funds provided under the Hill-Burton Act could be withdrawn from a hospital if it did not provide, at cost to itself, interpreter service for non-English speaking patients. This decision, and the ensuing monitoring by the Civil Rights Office, provided sufficient leverage for hospitals to adopt language interpretation requirements for all admissions, transfers, and treatment decisions and to secure adequately trained interpreters to provide direct services. This legal action, spurred by a coming together of community interests, helped to enable high-quality nursing and health care for vulnerable populations of newcomers.

Some of the information for this report was contributed by
Sherry Riddick, RN, MPH, director, Interpretation Programs, Central Seattle
Community Health Centers.

Program 4:   Community-Initiated Program
The Seattle Quilt Project, Seattle, Wash.

LySieng Ngo has been a professional medical interpreter for the Central Seattle Community Health Center since she arrived as a refugee from Cambodia in 1979. Born and raised in Cambodia, she had to hide her urban educated background during the Pol Pot years, 1975-79. As hardship turned to torture, she watched her pet dog die of starvation, faced the disappearance of her mother during an ordinary trip to town, lost her father to starvation, nursed the grandmother with whom she slept every night as a child through her death, lost two sisters and many others, while staving off intermittent sickness, hunger, and extreme weight loss. After the Pol Pot regime was ousted, she survived an arduous trek to Thailand and lived in a refugee camp. She did not know the whereabouts of other family members, but she later found out that two sisters were in Australia and an aunt and cousins were in France. A brother who had gone abroad to school before the Pol Pot era was in Seattle. LySieng also settled there as did many other Cambodians.

Because she had friends who worked for the U.S. Embassy in Phnom Phen, LySieng was one of the few Cambodians in Seattle who spoke English. She was quickly chosen by community clinics to provide interpreter services for the growing numbers of Cambodian patients. Over the years, physicians and nurse practitioners developed consultative relationships with Ms. Ngo and even referred patients to her for routine follow up support. The patients under her purview were those most recalcitrant to medical intervention, least connected to Seattle and the local community, and most sad and depressed. Ms. Ngo "stuck by them," empathizing with their plight—perhaps in part—because she herself was also suffering PTSD. Yet she did not know how to help them or herself through it. The clinic staff solidly supported her, a few becoming major sources of emotional support in her life. Once LySieng was so depressed she could do nothing but hide in a country cabin. She stayed up all night sewing a quilt. The next morning she felt much better. When she told the clinic staff about this experience, they told her about quilting bees, something that was new to her. So, in January 1993, LySieng asked if she could start one for her women clients at the clinic. Although there was no analogous tradition among Cambodian women, the quilt-making provided a reason for coming together and for relating, even nonverbally, with others, slowly coaxing the women out of their protective shells.

The women made several quilts, the first were used to decorate the clinic walls. Through this activity, the women found a way they could give something and found a way out of a dependent position in which they felt different from other Seattle people. They began talking about their recollections from Cambodia—they had not done so before even though they never forgot the past. They became more animated, and each began making her own quilts to sell. One woman who had secluded herself at home for 10 years used the money she earned from her quilts to buy plants for a garden. The first time she opened her door and saw them blooming she smiled. Her husband asked her why, but she wouldn't tell him because she thought he didn't care about flowers. Ever since she had cancer, he had insisted that she stay in the house all the time in order to avoid getting sick. But now she spends all day outside every day. Like her quilting friends, now her recent memory has come back and she has more interest in life.

In 1994, Ms. Ngo was awarded a Robert Wood Johnson Fellowship in Community Leadership because of her work at the clinic with Cambodian women. The original cohort of women are moving beyond quilting as their main endeavor, into gardening and studying English.

This self-help intervention was successful for many reasons, including, of course, the unusual character and dedication of Ms. Ngo. The clinic was her daytime home and became one for her clients. The clinic staff were her ever-ready support personally and professionally—her family on the job. They were partners in easing overwhelming depression into social activity, silent smiles, occasional humor, and a renewed pleasure in the moment.

Information about this program was contributed by Marjorie Muecke, RN, PhD, FAAN, program officer, the Ford Foundation.

Program 5:   Community-Initiated Program
CARACEN, San Francisco, Calif.

A multi-service center, the Central American Resource Center (CARECEN) of San Francisco opened its doors in 1986. Initially, CARECEN focused on providing legal services to those in need. A non-profit corporation, CARECEN receives support from 28 foundations, a staff of 30, and 135 active volunteers.

Most of the organization's bilingual staff are members of the Latino immigrant community. CARECEN serves primarily Latino immigrants, the homeless, and low-income communities of all nationalities. It strives to create programs which preserve, respect, and celebrate the culture of its community.

Among its programs, CARECEN offers three projects specifically for women. The Women's Wellness Clinic is held weekly at CARECEN's Celina Ramos Clinic for low-income and homeless communities. Women may either drop-in on Tuesdays or schedule an appointment for other days. Services include counseling, support groups, and basic gynecologic exams. In addition, the Women's Wellness Clinic offers health education on a range of topics such as breast self-examination, mental health, diet, and children's immunizations. Clients receive treatment as needed or are referred to the regular CARECEN clinic.

PASOS is a CARECEN project providing opportunities for a woman to succeed outside of college, which may not otherwise be possible at this time in her life. Participants are at-risk young women, usually single mothers, prostitutes, gang members, and so on who are willing to learn to be dental assistants, operate computers, and do general office management at the CARECEN site. These women have the opportunity to give back to their community by helping in the clinic and office for up to 1 year. At the same time, they receive an education and stipend.

JOVENES UNIDOS (Young Newcomers Project) serves girls and boys ages 8-17, providing in-school and after school education, recreation, and delinquency prevention. While some activities are coed, the project also runs activities exclusively for girls. Jovenes Unidos seeks to meet the special needs of newcomer girls from Nicaragua, El Salvador, Guatemala, and Mexico which include English-language and acculturation classes. The project includes support groups at five school sites each semester, as well as case-management services for girls and their families. The gender-specific activities foster an environment where girls work together to reinforce their cultural identity and self-esteem. The program offers the girls an oppotunity to develop their skills through learning styles specific to teen women— away from the pressures and distractions of co-educational activities. Services at the school site include: daily homework assistance and tutoring, nutrition and snacks, cultural arts, mental health counseling, computer training, all-girls sports activities, health education, journalism, dance and music classes, field trips, career exploration, family literacy, math and science, case management and mental health crisis intervention as needed, and community projects.

Information about this project was contributed by Sr. Petra Chavez of CARECEN.

Program 6:   Community-Initiated Program
Haitian Health Foundation, Miami, Fla.

In 1992, a group of Haitian-American health care professionals formed the Haitian Health Foundation to improve the South Florida's Haitian community's access to health care. Poor access is related to language difficulties, poverty, and lack of education. The foundation has received several small grants to support specific projects but has also accomplished considerable work on a voluntary basis. The first project was AIDS education for Haitian women and included an AIDS workshop at an elementary school, an AIDS education fair, and distribution of educational materials in Creole, including a clever calendar with cartoon-like teaching scenes. The program focused on teaching Haitian women to protect themselves and to work toward changing their partners' behavior.

The foundation also established a primary-care clinic in a Miami elementary school to serve 300 students and their parents. Staffed by volunteer Haitian nurses and physicians, the clinic is open 1 day a week and will soon be open on Saturdays as well. Clinic staff focus on disease prevention, early intervention, and health education—with home followup as necessary. The clinic staff offers medical (mainly adult), pediatric, dental, and mental health services as well as vision screening and referral. The clinic staff also teach hygiene, dental hygiene, nutrition, fire safety, and general safety. The foundation is currently opening a similar clinic in a local church.

The newest project is developing an organization of volunteer women within the Haitian community of Fort Lauderdale in collaboration with Haitian Outreach Partnership for Empowerment (HOPE). These women are sharing information on health problems and the associated risks affecting their lifestyles. They are working in partnership with schools, businesses, churches, health care providers, and the media to train a core of outreach workers. As they gain awareness and confidence, they will independently manage and maintain the project. The 7-week training sessions are taught in Creole and English by volunteer health professionals on such topics as immunizations, nutrition, tuberculosis, HIV/AIDS, breast self-examination, Pap-smear screening, and cardiopulmonary resuscitation. When the women complete the training, they are armed with culturally and linguistically appropriate pictographic pamphlets and a resource directory for making referrals.

The Haitian Health Foundation and HOPE have conducted four series of classes in a Baptist church, 50 women in each class. Women who attended the first two trainings helped to teach the second two series. So far, this effort has resulted in home visits for approximately 100 women. In addition, there is a monthly presentation to the Haitian community at large on topics similar to those in the trainings. There has been a tremendous response from women in the church as well as the community. The number of women reached by health education should multiply quickly, reaching to an ever-widening group of Haitian women. The program will be evaluated by master's level nursing students from Florida Atlantic University.

Information about this foundation was contributed by Jessie Colin, RN, MS, PhD candidate, one of the originators and active teachers.

Program 7: **Nurse-Initiated Program**
Mid-East S.I.H.A. Project, San Francisco, Calif.

The Mid-East Study of Immigration, Health, and Adjustment (S.I.H.A.) Project was established in an office in the Department of Mental Health, Community and Adminstrative Nursing (now Community Health Systems) at the University of California, San Francisco in 1982, based on several years of consultation requests from health care professionals in reference to Middle-Eastern immigrant clients.

The threefold purpose of the project is research, education, and service. The project has provided a structure for studies of ethnic identity, immigration and health, Arab families' care of children, first generation Jordanian adolescents, postpartum and birth control practices among Arab women, marital strains related to immigration, and Lebanese immigrants' conceptions of health. Educational activities include encouraging doctoral students in nursing and anthropology to study or practice with Middle-Eastern populations and in-service and continuing education for health professionals in reference to health issues and cultural patterns.

Service to Middle-Eastern immigrants and to health and social service personnel who work with them include a 1-day-a-week clinic in which project members are available to work with clients around a variety of issues. The intent is not to provide new health care services, but to complement existing services with culturally sensitive client advocacy, health education, counseling, referral, and consultation with clients' regular health care providers.

Project members from Egypt, Jordan, Iraq, Iran, Israel, and the United States work on a voluntary basis, sharing responsibilities depending on availability and requisite skills for the task. The project's staff has provided information, referral, physical and psychological assessment, patient advocacy, counseling, translation and cultural interpretation, health education, and consultation to health care professionals. The staff has also compiled a resource guide for services available in the San Francisco Bay Area and developed a health-assessment tool.

Since the clinic began, the bulk of the service has been to clients needing psychiatric and mental health services, and the project's members have done assessments, counseling, and arranging for psychiatric hospitalization when necessary. Cultural and language interpreters have been provided who work closely with mental health personnel, sometimes as co-therapists. The project's staff also does a lot of consultation in reference to hospitalized patients who are monolingual in Arabic or Farsi, at the request of health professionals who know little about Middle-Eastern cultures. Clients include Palestinian, Jordanian, Lebanese, Armenian, Yemeni, Iraqi, Iranian, and Saudi immigrants.

Women's Health-Education Program. This health promotion program was developed to reach immigrant women in the Arab community. Called "Being Healthy, Thinking Healthy, Staying Healthy," the program consisted of eight 90-minute workshops: handling life as an immigrant, maintaining child health and safety, raising adolescents, finding a job, promoting good nutrition with Arab foods, menopause, women's self-care, and AIDS prevention.

The U.S. Arab population is heterogeneous and has not been accurately counted in the census, so key informants, community forums, surveys, and ethnographic procedures were used to obtain information about health needs and health education topics for the community. Program planning was undertaken through weekly meetings with the presidents of five Arab women's organizations to obtain input on community needs. The following strategies proved essential to success: (a) enhancing trust, (b) acknowledging the diversity of the community without aligning with any one segment, and (c) considering current events in the countries of the immigrant's origin.

Community women were active participants in choosing topics, translating, typing, and distributing brochures and health education materials, booking space for workshops, organizing transportation, babysitting, inviting friends, and evaluating the program. Speakers were oriented before their sessions to the workshop goals and audience. Following each workshop, the project coordinator telephoned the organization's spokeswomen for their reactions and suggestions for change. Participants completed evaluation forms on a regular basis.

Information about this program was contributed by Afaf Meleis, RN, PhD, FAAN, director, and Juliene Lipson, RN, PhD, FAAN, codirector.

References

Arab women immigrants' health education. (1994). Program notes: Health education in practice. **Health Education Quarterly 21(1)**, 7-8.

Meleis, A.I., & Lipson J.G. (1993). Mid-East SIHA - A primary health care center. In M. J. Kim, (Ed.), Primary Health Care: Nurses Lead the Way—A Global Perspective (pp. 19-24). AACN and WHO Regional Office of the American Pan American Health Organization.

Meleis, A.I., Omidian P. A., & Lipson, J.G. (1993). Women's health status in the United States: An immigrant women's project. In B. J. McElmurry, K. F. Norr, & R. S. Parker (Eds.), **Women's health and development: A global challenge** (pp. 163-181). Boston: Jones and Bartlett.

Program 8:   Nurse-Initiated Program
<u>Afghan Health Education Project</u>,
Fremont, Calif.

The Afghan Health Education Project (AHEP) was developed with funding by the Health Education—Risk Reduction Program (HE-RR), State of California Department of Health Services, Health Promotion Section. The goals of this contract were to develop an ethnic community coalition, conduct a community health assessment, and determine needs for language and culturally appropriate health education to help reduce the risks of chronic diseases and problems outlined in Healthy People 2000.

Meeting in Fremont, with a large population of Afghan refugees, the project was guided by a steering committee of nine members—six Afghans, three Americans—which met weekly over the 16 months of funding. The assessment consisted of an exploratory telephone survey, seven community meetings, and a survey of 196 families. At the end of the funding period AHEP held the first Afghan Community Health Fair. Despite lack of success in obtaining further funding, the Afghan community's appetite for health education was whetted and those involved in the project have continued to look for opportunities to continue informal health education.

One such opportunity presented itself when Cathy Bernstein, a UCSF master's student, offered to teach a breast self-exam class to Afghan women. Cathy, studying to be a nurse practitioner specializing in women's health, read all the available literature on Afghan refugees and their culture and prepared carefully. The two women Afghan Health Education Project steering committee members invited many women and arranged the time and place for the class. They drove the women to the meeting, introduced everyone, brought refreshments appropriate for Norooz (Afghan New Year), and reinforced the teaching.

About 12 women attended, three of whom were elderly and wore traditional clothing and head scarfs. The chairs were set in a circle and the class was videotaped so that other women could learn from it as well. However, only Cathy and Dr. Maryam were shown because the other women seemed uncomfortable about being videotaped.

The format was informal, with many side conversations in Dari and Pashto as is typical of an Afghan gathering, yet the women were paying attention. Two women left the class early to pick up their children from school and brought them back to the class. One older woman placed her jacket on the floor in a corner of the room and kneeled to pray at the appropriate time.

Cathy presented information in English, drawing on paper, which may have been less threatening than showing actual photographs of breasts. Dr. Maryam, a physician not yet licensed to practice medicine in the United States, interpreted, explained, and taught. There were no written materials in Dari, but Cathy explained the pictures on handouts written in English. The older women looked particularly interested; most likely, having had no formal education, they did not know the anatomy and physiology of their breasts. They were very interested in touching and practicing examinations on the breast models. The women asked several clinical questions; for example, one woman had questions about painful cysts and had not been helped by three doctors she had consulted. Cathy suggested calling the UCSF breast-health center. A young woman asked about the risk of developing breast cancer. The older women had everyone howling with laughter, making jokes when Cathy suggested husbands helping with breast exam— "if the husband does the exam, he will want to do it every day." The women also thought it would be very strange to ask a friend to call and remind them to do it each month, as well as looking in the mirror at themselves naked.

Cathy and Dr. Maryam followed up by calling each woman after 2 months to see if she was doing breast self-examination. After several weeks, those who had attended told the organizers how much they had enjoyed and learned from the class and asked when there would be other classes on women's health.

While AHEP is no longer funded, an important offshoot of the community-health assessment and emphasis on health education was that women steering committee members helped to develop the Afghan Women Association International which has continued to be very active in health related community activities. Examples are the second Afghan community health fair, health education classes, and a support group for Afghan women.

Information about this program was contributed by Juliene Lipson,
former director, Afghan Health Education Project.

Reference

Lipson, J. G., Hosseini, T., Kabir, S., Omidian, P., & Edmonston, F. (1995). Health issues among Afghan women in California. **Health Care for Women International, 16**, 279-286.

Program 9:   Nurse-Initiated Program
After-school programs for Vietnamese Children, Chicago, Ill.

Having had some volunteer experience in teaching and providing primary health care to hill tribe peoples in northern Thailand, Patricia Fox, RN, PhD, has continued relating to groups from Southeast Asia in the United States. As a faculty member in Public Health Nursing at the College of Nursing, University of Illinois, Chicago, she and Julia Cowell, RNC, PhD, are conducting an intervention study in Chicago of children and their mothers who resettled in this country as refugees. They have studied whether and how the children's experience with violence before coming to the United

States might affect their current lives. Although they found rates of depression higher than for other Americans in both the children and their mothers, the rates were not related to premigration experiences. Instead, the researchers attributed the high rates to the challenges of adaptation to a new environment, in particular to an urban environment fraught with poverty, crime, and neglect.

Fox and her colleagues have taken action to address their findings. In collaboration with the local Cambodian Association and the Vietnamese Association of Illinois, they secured funding to develop after-school programs for children from Cambodia and Vietnam in neighborhood elementary schools. Bilingual education teachers and school nurses conduct the programs and also visit the children's mothers in their homes to assess their needs, provide support, and link them to community resources. Fox and Cowell are in the process of evaluating the program in order to identify successful approaches that might be replicated.

Information about this program was contributed by
Patricia Fox, College of Nursing, University of Illinois at Chicago.

References

Fox, P. G., Cowell, J., & Montgomery, A. (1994). The effects of violence on health and adjustment of Southeast Asian refugee children: An integrative review. **Public Health Nursing, 11**, 195-201.

Fox, P. G., Cowell, J. M., & Johnson, M. (1995). The effects of family disruption on Southeast Asian refugee women: Implications for international nursing. **International Nursing Review, 42**, 27-30.

Fox, P. G., Cowell, J. M., & Montgomery, A. (1996). Premigration violence experience of Southeast Asian refugee children in the United States. **International Journal of Psychiatric Nursing Research, 2**, 211-223.

Program 10: Association-Initiated Program
Haitian American Nurses Association of Florida, Miami, Fla.

The Haitian American Nurses Association of Florida, Inc. (HANA), in existence for 11 years, provides health education to the Haitian community in Miami. While community outreach is not specifically targeted to women in Haitian culture, women oversee the health and welfare of the entire family. Most attendees at HANA's health programs are women, who then take information home and implement the care needed.

HANA does community outreach through a variety of means and settings. Most outreach efforts are centered in Miami's Little Haiti. Some examples include hypertension screening and education in churches, children's immunizations and physical examinations in schools, HIV Prevention Day, blood pressure screening and education at Haitian Roots and Culture festivals, and various flea-market booths.

At the flea markets, members used the loudspeaker to announce the booth and the next community health fair and attracted people through music and offering free gifts. HANA's members provided health education literature in Creole, English, and Spanish and talked with women about breast cancer and with men about prostate cancer.

HANA organizes community health fairs four times a year, using a multi-disciplinary approach. Members work with physicians, social workers, and dieticians to provide culturally sensitive education and care. Services include diabetes education, hypertension screening and education, AIDS education, and immunization for preschool children. Programs specific to women include breast cancer screening through a cancer prevention Mobile Unit (mammograms) and breast self-exam classes in a school classroom.

HANA provides health education programs outside of Little Haiti through radio broadcasts on WKAT 1320 AM, the most popular radio station among Haitians. These programs are presented whenever the budget permits doing so or when a local Haitian community-oriented group provides the opportunity. Radio programs emphasize education and reeducation with messages such as the following: "Diabetes and hypertension are chronic diseases requiring long term management, not a one-shot treatment"; "Do not share your medication with others who have the same diagnosis"; "Tell your physician what home remedies you are taking when he prescribes medication."

HANA's members believe that culturally sensitive teaching is most effective, and that every little bit helps. Therefore, members creatively use every existing opportunity and also develop new efforts to help the Haitian community learn about and improve health.

Information about this exemplar was provided by
Ghislaine Paperwalla, president, HANA.

APPENDIX

B

Policy Recommendations

1. Aid to immigrants must be restored and expanded in order to assure that women have timely access to needed health care services regardless of legal status. A national health program should be implemented that offers universal access to health care regardless of legal status.

2. Administrative rules and regulations should be developed to broaden the current type of data collected at federal and state levels so that ethnic and racial subgroups are listed.

3. Private foundations, state and local governments, and state and local organizations should continue to support demonstration projects and their linkages with comprehensive, integrated health delivery systems.

4. Private foundations, state and local governments, and state and local organizations should assist and support the development of self-help groups.

5. Many special committees and interest groups on women's health and international health exist within organized nursing. These interest groups should join forces for concentrated developmental work over time on knowledge, skill, and action that make such groups successful and recognized champions of immigrant women's health.

6. Nursing organizations should cooperate and work proactively with other organizations to develop a focused policy-informing strategy and a research agenda on women, health, and poverty.

7. Members of nursing organizations should address how they might work with other appropriate groups to ensure that students in all health professions are introduced to explicit ways of developing appropriate culturally sensitive interventions and have related experiences in clinical and community settings to reinforce the learning.

8. Members of nursing organizations should address how they might facilitate identification and dissemination of strategies that work for the collecting and analyzing of health-status data at local levels.

9. Members of nursing organizations should address how they might facilitate the identification and dissemination of health and human service programs that work.

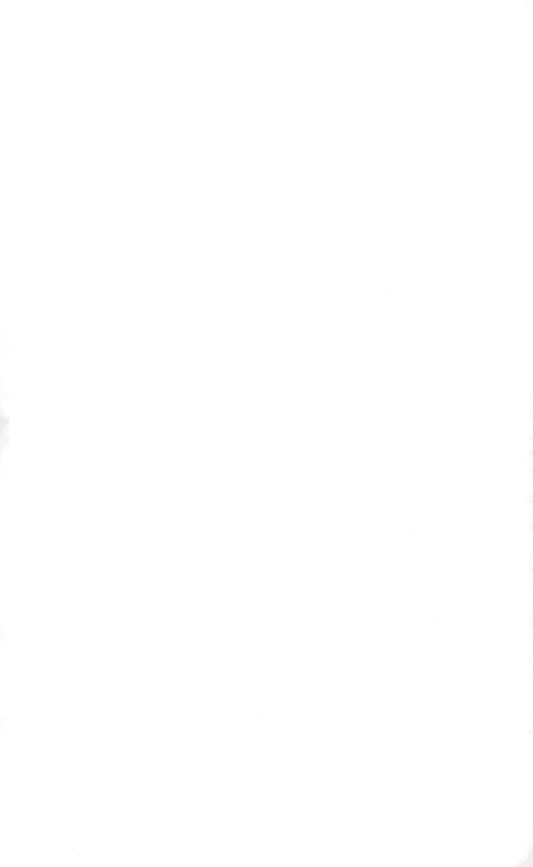